# ...CKY DOG
# WEIGHT LOSS PLAN

## Vicky Marshall

### The Mammoth Publishing Company

Copyright 2015 by Vicky Marshall

Printed in the United Kingdom
First Edition

All rights reserved; no part of this publication may be reproduced, stored in a retrieval system, or transmitted in any form or by any means, electronic, mechanical, photocopying, recording or otherwise without the prior written permission of the publisher. This book is sold subject to the condition that it shall not, by way of trade or otherwise, be lent, re-sold, hired out, or otherwise circulated without the publisher's prior consent in any form of binding or cover other than that in which it is published.

First published in 2015
The Mammoth Publishing Company
An imprint of Wentworth Publishing Limited
17 Fleet Street, London EC4 Y1AA
Telephone 020 7353 7300
Web: www.mammothpublishing.com
ISBN: 978-0-9570753-1-3

For my darling family
Gary, James, Kate & Harry
...and our own 'Lucky Dogs'
Rudi-Doodle and Fletcher.

## THE LUCKY DOG WEIGHT LOSS PLAN

### Contents

|     | | |
| --- | --- | --- |
|  | Foreword by Richard Allport BVet Med. Vet MFHom MRCVS | *9* |
| 1. | How to transform your dog's weight with a simple change of diet | *15* |
| 2. | A bluffer's guide to the Lucky Dog Diet | *23* |
| 3. | Why dogs are wrestling with their weight for the first time in 4 million years | *31* |
| 4. | The Lucky Dog Diet! | *41* |
| 5. | Extra tips and advice | *59* |
| 6. | Making the switch to the Lucky Dog Diet | *71* |
| 7. | Why wolves and wild dogs never get fat (even when there is plenty of food around) | *79* |
| 8. | Give a dog a bone | *89* |
| 9. | The unpalatable truth about modern dog food | *97* |
| 10. | A chapter about something no one likes to mention | *109* |
| 11. | Myth buster! | *115* |
| 12. | What to do once your dog reaches his or her target weight | *123* |
| 13. | Safe weight loss for sick and poorly dogs | *131* |
| 14. | The Lucky Dog Diet is approved and supported by these leading vets | *161* |
| 15. | More help if you need it | *169* |
|  | Further reading | *179* |

# FOREWORD
## BY RICHARD ALLPORT
## BVET MED. VET MFHOM
## MRCVS

## FOREWORD

## **FOREWORD**

When I qualified as a vet in 1973 and was therefore entitled to put the letters MRCVS (Member of the Royal College of Veterinary Surgeons) after my name, the world was a very different place, and veterinary practice was a very different world.

If you were sitting in the waiting room of your local vet in 1973 you would have noticed two striking differences compared with sitting in the waiting room of your vet today. Firstly, the sales area (had there been one) was not packed from floor to ceiling with pet food. Secondly, there were very few obese dogs amongst the throng of pets waiting to see the vet.

Over the years, and over the last couple of decades in particular, there has been a phenomenal growth in the number of obese dogs amongst the canine population. Why is this so? It may be true that some dogs are getting insufficient exercise, but the increase in obesity has mirrored the increase in the feeding of high carbohydrate, low quality protein, processed diets. I don't believe this can be a coincidence.

Dogs in the seventies were mainly fed on scraps, leftovers, bones and cheap meat and offal from the local butcher. There were few dog treats available and most dogs had plenty of walks and runs. Obesity was rare. Dogs today are commonly fed on kibble, a form of dried food that is high in fats (to give it some taste) and in carbohydrates, and low in high quality protein. Essentially, this is junk food for dogs. Most canned foods are little better, some containing as little as three or four per cent real meat. There is a plethora of dog treats on the market. And obesity is common.

Dogs are carnivores. They have evolved to eat meat, offal, raw bones and vegetables. Dogs are social animals. They are designed to have lots of play and interaction with other dogs and with their human companions. If they eat what they have evolved to eat and are given the physical and mental stimulation they need, they will not get overweight. It's as simple as that.

One caveat – some medical conditions, such as hypothyroidism, Cushing's disease, diabetes and others, can cause a dog to become overweight. Hypothyroidism (an underactive thyroid) is often hard to diagnose, and there are probably quite a number of obese dogs that have an underlying thyroid imbalance.

If your dog is becoming obese, and does not have a medical condition that may be causing the weight gain, what can you do about it? Your local vet may well have a weight control clinic. You can take your dog for a regular weigh in, and will be given advice about nutrition by a practice nurse, who will probably have a qualification in canine nutrition. Should you enquire whence this qualification came, it will almost certainly be a certificate or diploma granted by one of the major pet food manufacturers. For instance, many veterinary nurses are 'Hills Pet Nutrition Advisers'. Hills is a multinational conglomerate that sells a range of processed foods, especially kibbles, and sponsors many veterinary meetings and advertises heavily to the veterinary profession.

There are several other multinationals that do much the same. Some provide free food to veterinary colleges and to animal charities, and some have actually paid the salaries of vets who lecture students on nutrition at veterinary colleges.

It seems unlikely that a major pet food company can train a veterinary nurse in nutrition without just a smidgeon of bias towards their own products. Products which are likely to be expensive and, in my view, entirely unnecessary 'therapeutic' weight reduction diet foods.

Rather than wasting your time, energy and money on visits to weight control clinics and pointless diets, read the following pages instead. Vicky Marshall explains clearly and straightforwardly what dogs should be eating, how their digestive systems work, why they can become obese, and how to get them back on track if they are getting overweight.

Lucky indeed is the dog that benefits from the wisdom and common sense of the Lucky Dog Diet.

Richard Allport<br>
BVet Med. Vet MFHom MRCVS

# 1.
# HOW TO TRANSFORM YOUR DOG'S WEIGHT WITH A SIMPLE CHANGE OF DIET

# ONE

The old ways are sometimes the best ways. A hundred years ago, even fifty years ago, very few dogs had weight issues. Whatever they were doing or being fed it wasn't affecting their collar sizes or their waistlines. Today, however, approximately half of British dogs are either overweight or obese.

What has happened to bring about this change?

Certainly, it doesn't help that society as a whole has become more sedentary or that legislation means that a dog can no longer get extra exercise by roaming freely around the neighbourhood where he or she lives.

It is possible, too, that dogs have become more persuasive when asking for extra food and treats.

However, I am certain, based on my experience of feeding several thousand dogs a month, that the main cause is modern dog food. Modern dog food is high in simple carbohydrate, low in protein and full of harmful fats – the perfect recipe if you want to push a dog's weight up.

Indeed, it is no coincidence that within a few years of the formula being developed, a growing number of dogs began to pile on the pounds.

Thankfully, the effects of modern dog food are quickly reversed. If there is a dog in your life who isn't quite as slim or svelte as you would like, the solution is straightforward. All you have to do is feed your four-legged family member a more traditional, more natural diet. The same sort of diet, in fact, that our great-grandparents fed to their dogs.

Implementing such a diet is simplicity itself, which is why this book is so short! Moreover, not only will your dog adore the change, but also his or her excess weight will fall away as if by magic. This will bring about another benefit: better health. All the research indicates that dogs who are the correct weight suffer less illness and disease.

I developed the Lucky Dog Weight Loss Plan (aka the Lucky Dog Diet) through observation and experiment but my findings reflect extensive scientific research. The predominant components of the Lucky Dog Diet are high protein, low carbohydrate and the right quantity of 'good' fat. It can take as little as two weeks for an overweight dog to achieve its target weight on this diet, although I generally suggest that you don't rush the process and allow between 60 and 90 days, or longer. One of the many benefits of the diet is that it leads to the loss of fat, not muscle mass, which is much healthier for your dog. Independent research, incidentally, has shown that the two main components of the Lucky Dog Diet leave dogs feeling 'fuller' than a wide range of alternative ingredients.

If you read this book through to the end you will find a chapter about my own business: Honey's Real Dog Food. We have a policy at Honey's of providing free diet and health advice to anyone who contacts us, even if they never intend to become a customer. Please do get in touch if we can be of any assistance. We have a special team that looks after poorly and/or overweight dogs.

Finally, you will notice that throughout this book I make reference to 'biologically appropriate food' and you may wonder what I mean by this. Every species on earth needs to eat a biologically appropriate diet. Otherwise it will become ill and/or die. Pandas, for example, must eat bamboo. Dogs, as I will be explaining, share the identical digestive system to the grey wolf (not so surprising given that they are so closely related they can interbreed) and flourish on the same diet. It is thanks to this diet that you never, ever see an overweight wolf, no matter how much he or she eats. That's how good the Lucky Dog Diet is!

## WHEN TO SEEK EXPERIENCED HELP

There are circumstances when a switch to the Lucky Dog Diet should only be undertaken with experienced guidance. Dogs that have recently undergone bowel surgery or chemotherapy or that have a compromised immune system can all benefit from the Lucky Dog Diet but may need a special diet. Also, pregnant dogs and new mums will have special nutritional needs. Please do contact us at Honey's for free advice (you don't have to be a customer) or consult a vet or other professional with relevant expertise (see chapter 14 for a list of vets who have approved and support the Lucky Dog Diet).

# EXPLODING THE 'HIGH PROTEIN' MYTH

I refer to the Lucky Dog Diet as being a 'high protein, low carbohydrate diet incorporating the correct balance of "good" fats'.

Because modern, processed dog food has very low levels of very poor quality protein (often from vegetable sources, that dogs can't absorb), manufacturers have done their best to persuade everyone that protein is not good for a dog.

In fact, high quality, animal protein is exactly what your dog needs to thrive.

# HOW MUCH PROTEIN?

The secret is to give your dog the same levels that he or she would enjoy if they decided, as a result of seeing too many disaster movies, to leave home and become self-sufficient survivalists, living in the wilderness and fending for themselves.

This would vary from meal to meal, of course, as I'll explain later on.

The real point I want to make now is that the natural level of protein found in the diet I am recommending is perfect for your dog.

# 2.
# A BLUFFER'S GUIDE TO THE LUCKY DOG DIET

## TWO

Pressed for time but keen to understand the basics of the Lucky Dog Diet? Here is a summary of all the main points made in this book:

### *Why some dogs can't help piling on the pounds*

As many as half the dogs in the UK are either overweight or obese. Why? Lack of exercise plays a role, but the main reason is modern dog food. Over the last few decades manufacturers have switched to a formula that is making it difficult for dogs to stay trim, namely: low levels of protein, high levels of simple carbohydrate and an excess of unhealthy fats. Yes, lots of dogs would benefit from additional exercise. Yes, there are dogs who, like Oscar Wilde, can resist anything but temptation (especially if the temptation comes in the form of treats and titbits). But the underlying problem is that modern dog food is fattening.

### *The quick, easy and pleasurable way for dogs to lose weight*

The quick, easy and pleasurable way for dogs to lose weight is to switch from modern, processed dog food to the same sort of diet they ate before the dog food manufacturers grew to dominate the market. Such a diet is high in natural protein, low in carbohydrate and includes the right balance of 'good' fats. It's the same diet that wolves eat in the wild. This is not a co-incidence! Dogs and wolves are so closely related that they can interbreed and possess identical digestive systems. Once dogs switch to a traditional, natural diet the weight falls off them, as if by magic. Best of all, they really love the food because it is full of extra flavour and texture.

## Readily available ingredients

The Lucky Dog Diet requires very little preparation (literally a couple of minutes a day), the instructions are simple and all the ingredients you need are available from your supermarket or butcher. The main ingredients may surprise you – raw meat, raw bone and fresh vegetables – but when you think about what wolves and dogs eat in the wild, the rationale for the diet becomes apparent. There's a short, scientific explanation about why this diet is so good for your dog below and more on the subject later on in the book. The diet is suitable for any dog. What's more, you'll notice that the Lucky Dog Diet doesn't require you to count calories. This is because the amount of food you feed your dog is based on his or her weight. Another thing, this diet leads to loss of unnecessary fat and not valuable muscle mass.

## How to speed things up

The Lucky Dog Diet is much, much more effective when accompanied by an exercise programme. The best option is to get your dog out and about, but if this really isn't feasible, don't worry. There are ways of increasing the amount of exercise your dog receives without you having to leave home. For example, if you put a little bit of food into a Kong (a type of rubber toy) and play a game of fetch your dog will burn a surprising amount of calories. Exercise will improve your dog's health, as well as his or her waistline, so it would be better to incorporate it into the Lucky Dog Diet. Still, just changing your dog's diet will make a massive difference.

## Long-term benefits of the Lucky Dog Diet

Having slimmed your dog down to the correct weight using the Lucky Dog Diet there is every reason to carry on feeding him or her the same diet. As those who have switched their dogs to a natural diet will testify, the results can be amazing. Benefits include a glossy coat, healthy skin, lean muscle tone, robust immune system, sweet-smelling breath, healthy teeth and gums, increased energy, better digestion and a strong heart. Dogs eating a natural diet can be expected to live longer and to suffer less illness and disease.

## Why the Lucky Dog Diet is so effective

The reason why the Lucky Dog Diet is so effective is that it features what is generally referred to as a 'biologically appropriate' food. What does this mean? Each creature on earth needs a specific range of foods to survive and prosper. Otherwise, it will get ill and may (if the diet is really inappropriate) die. For the first 4 million years of dogs' existence on earth they certainly didn't eat canned food or kibble. Four million years? Yes, that's how long wolves have been around, and dogs and wolves are classified as the same species. When wolves were domesticated (around 8,000 to 20,000 years ago), we humans changed their outer appearance through breeding, but not their internal organs or digestive systems.

## In the wild, dogs eat prey and not much else

Dogs are carnivores (they do need a bit of herbage and if push comes to shove can survive on it) as even a cursory glance at their anatomy reveals. Like other predatory mammals, they have powerful muscles, fused wrist bones and a cardiovascular system that supports both sprinting and endurance. And there's a reason why you don't want to get bitten by a dog: their mouths are positive Swiss Army knives, with four kinds of exceedingly sharp teeth. Leave them to their own devices and they will eat small birds and beasts (rabbits, mice, squirrels &c.) and a share of larger prey (sheep, deer, boar &c.). What's more, they eat the whole animal, including its bones.

## Canine digestion is nothing like human digestion

Dogs have no digestive enzymes in their saliva (unlike humans) and very large, expandable stomachs (they can eat 5% of their bodyweight at a single sitting, which would be like someone who weighs 10 stone eating seven pounds of food in one go) not to mention indescribably strong stomach acids (strong enough to burn your fingers). Their digestive system is designed so that they can tear off chunks of raw meat, crunch up raw bones and swallow the lot whole. The lack of digestive enzymes in their saliva and their inability to move their jaws from side to side (necessary to grinding food) is why they gulp everything down. The entire digestive process takes place in their stomach.

## Give a dog a bone

In the wild, up to a third of a dog's nutrition (including calcium, magnesium, complex fats and vitamins) may come from bones. Bones keep their teeth and gums clean (it has been proven that dogs with healthy teeth live longer) and exercise their upper body and jaw. Providing the bones are raw (cooked bones can splinter) and certain basic rules are observed (all revealed in chapter 8!), they are 100% safe for dogs to eat.

## What else is wrong with modern, processed dog food?

I have already explained how modern, processed dog food is contributing to our dogs' weight issues. But it has other problems with it as well:

- It is cooked. Cooking destroys 70% of the nutritional value of the food from a dog's perspective and makes it exceedingly difficult to digest.

- It can contain inappropriate and damaging chemicals (binders, colouring, preservatives and other additives). These may be absorbed through the bowel wall and transported to other organs, with a range of harmful effects.
- The quality of the ingredients is usually poor. Even expensive dog food often has very, very low-quality ingredients.
- Most dog foods contain a high percentage of grain (including rice), which is unsuitable for the canine digestive system and causes allergies.
- It generally fails to clean the dog's teeth and gums, allowing plaque to build up. This gives rise to periodontal disease and worse.

# 3.
# WHY DOGS ARE WRESTLING WITH THEIR WEIGHT FOR THE FIRST TIME IN FOUR MILLION YEARS

THE FIRST TIME IN FOUR MILLION YEARS

## THREE

British dogs are getting heavier. The most recent research into this was conducted by the Pet Food Manufacturers Association (PFMA), which found that 45 out of every 100 dogs were either overweight or obese, a substantial increase on the previous survey. The organisation called upon pet owners to 'resist overfeeding and excessive treating'.

There is an irony to the PFMA's interest in this area as many of their members, being dog food manufacturers, could be considered part of the problem, not part of the solution. Modern dog food, with its lack of protein, high level of carbohydrates and unhealthy fats, is the single most important reason why our canine companions are becoming chubbier.

Moreover, manufacturers, never being slow to see a business opportunity, have now developed special 'weight loss' dog foods to correct a situation largely of their own making. These diet foods tend to be packed with crude fibre (such as beet pulp or peanut shells), which has the effect of filling a dog up without offering it any nutrition whatsoever.

### *Nature knows best*

Before I say another word, what dog food manufacturers are trying to do, in their warped way, is replicate a natural diet using inexpensive and often inappropriate ingredients. Modern dog food is highly processed and, almost without exception, utilises poor quality ingredients, which through methods such as cooking and extrusion, have lost most of whatever nutritional value they may ever have contained. What we are talking about is junk food for dogs. The best way for any species (including humans) to get their nutrition is in its most natural form.

## What dogs eat when given the choice

The best way to understand the shortcomings of modern, processed dog food is to compare it with a dog's biologically appropriate diet (the food it must have to optimise its health). Happily, we have two ways of knowing what this is. Firstly, there has been a lot of research into what wild dogs (such as the dingoes in Australia) eat when they have complete freedom of choice. Secondly, domesticated dogs and wolves have the identical digestive systems from their teeth to – ahem – their tails. As they are the same species, this isn't so surprising, and it provides scientific proof as to why they should be eating the same diet.

What do wild dogs and wolves eat? Small and medium sized prey animals such as mice, voles, rabbits, birds and – where available – fish. They consume every bit of the animal, too, including the bones (which supply about a third of their nutritional requirements) and the stomach contents. They also scavenge, eating a wide variety of grasses, herbs, vegetables and fruits as well as less appetising things such as faeces.

### WHY YOUR DOG'S WEIGHT IS SUCH A BIG ISSUE

Does it really matter if your dog is carrying a little extra weight? If you care about your dog's health then the answer is yes. Excess weight will reduce your dog's life expectancy and will make him or her prone to all sorts of serious health problems including (but not only) joint disease, arthritis, heart disease, hypertension, respiratory problems, asthma, pancreatitis, diabetes, liver disease, skin issues, cancer and a compromised immune system.

## An analysis of a dog's natural diet

A very clever canine nutrition expert called Steve Brown has analysed what wild dogs and wolves eat in order to ascertain what domesticated dogs require. After extracting the water (in other words on a 'dry matter' basis) he found that the dog's natural diet consists of:

- 49% protein
- 44% fat
- 6% carbohydrate

By the way, although 44% of the calories come from fat, in terms of volume of food it only accounts for around 6% of the diet. This is because fat is calorie rich.

## Modern, processed dog food doesn't stack up that well

How does modern, processed dog food stack up when compared to a dog's natural diet? As the law allows manufacturers to present the ingredients they use in a very misleading way that is difficult to answer. For example, they can hide the percentage of carbohydrates and disguise the volume and type of fat. However, my own research suggests the following averages:

|  | Protein | Fat | Carbohydrate |
| --- | --- | --- | --- |
| Natural or wild diet | 49% | 44% | 6% |
| Dry food i.e. kibble | 27% | 30% | 43% |
| Canned food | 32% | 58% | 10% |

You'll notice that modern dog food is low in protein and high in carbohydrate. This is the opposite of a dog's natural diet and also contrary to all the scientific research regarding weight loss (which I will come on to in a moment). The fat content is low or high depending on whether you feed kibble or canned food, but either way it is harmful as manufacturers use inappropriate and unhealthy fat.

## The importance of protein

Why is the amount of protein in your dog's diet so important? And does it matter what the source of that protein is?

Protein is what your dog needs to form healthy cells, organs, protective tissue, hormones, enzymes, tendons and ligaments. It is essential for a good immune system and the mainstay of a wolf or wild dog's natural diet, accounting for around 90% of what it eats and providing around half the calories it requires. Research published in 2010 shows that a high-protein diet has the additional advantage of making a dog feel 'fuller'.

There is protein and protein! In a natural diet it comes almost completely from animal sources (meat and fish) which, unlike the vast majority of plants, contain the right balance of amino acids as well as a complete range of protein-type nutrients (for example, taurine and carnitine).

The protein in modern, processed dog food has various drawbacks. To begin with, the main constituent of protein, amino acids, are altered and can be destroyed by heat. It has, of course, been cooked. Even if the proteins survive the rendering process (when they are, essentially, boiled for a long period of time) they are of low quality, being from factory farmed animals. Also, some modern dog food relies on lesser, plant-based proteins.

The scientific evidence is clear: dogs need the protein supplied by a natural, raw diet.

## The importance of fat

Fats break down into three different types: saturated fats, monounsaturated fats and polyunsaturated fats. In their natural state in animals these

## WHAT THE EXPERTS SAY ABOUT PROTEIN

'Research shows that a high-protein, low-carbohydrate diet is the safest and most effective weight loss program for dogs,' say Jean Hofve DVM and Dr Celeste Yarnall, authors of *Paleo Dog*.

'Protein,' says Dr Lew Olson, author of *Raw and Natural Nutrition for Dogs*, 'is a dog's best friend.' She goes on to point out that: 'Recent studies have confirmed that a high level of protein is not just beneficial, but necessary for dogs of all ages.'

'Protein,' according to Steve Brown, author of *Unlocking the Canine Ancestral Diet*, 'provided 49% of the calories in the dog's ancestral diet, our gold standard.'

'Protein,' says Dr Karen Becker, author of *Real Food for Healthy Dogs and Cats*, 'is the foundation of the diet of a carnivore, necessary for the formation of healthy cells, enzymes, hormones, ligaments, tendons, organs and protective tissue. Next to water, it makes up the majority of our pet's body weight.'

'To maximize our pets' health,' says Dr Ian Billinghurst, author of *The BARF Diet: Raw Feeding for Dogs and Cats using Evolutionary Methods* (and other titles), 'we should supply our pets with protein that mimics the protein eaten by their wild ancestors.'

come from muscle meat, storage fat, bone marrow and organ fat. By feeding your dog different types of meat you make sure that he or she receives the right quantity of 'good' fats in their most natural state.

Fat is a vital part of your dog's diet. First and foremost, fat produces energy. The right sorts of fats are necessary for the absorption of fat-soluble vitamins. Additionally, they protect the nerve fibres in the body, provide protection from the cold, and are the ideal source of essential fatty acids. They are anti-inflammatory, too. The most important fatty acids for a dog are omega-6 and omega-3.

The fats you serve your dog should be fresh. Rancid and poor quality fats can really harm dogs, robbing them of essential fatty acids. The fat used in modern, processed dog food is of the poorest quality imaginable and comes from a variety of sources including the waste fat left over from fast food businesses. It has almost no nutritional value and is the single most important reason why dogs put on weight. Where extra fats (such as fish oils, a vital source of Omegas) are added to factory produced dog food they generally turn rancid by the time the food is eaten. This is because as soon as fat comes into contact with air it starts to oxidise. The more rancid a fat, the less valuable it is as it will have the effect of reducing the nutritional value of the protein, vitamins and antioxidants so necessary to your dog's health.

So, the rules with fat are (a) you must avoid the damaging fats in modern, processed dog food, (b) even though a dog may be trying to lose weight you shouldn't cut out fat completely, only reduce the quantity.

## *The problem with carbohydrates*

What is wrong with feeding a dog carbohydrates? Simple carbohydrates (such as rice, barley and oats) increase blood sugar, stimulate the production of pre-inflammatory hormones and (in plain English) play merry hell with a dog's immune system.

There is another problem, which is that dogs lack the digestive system required to convert most carbohydrates into a form they can actually use. Modern, processed dog food is very high in carbohydrates and the worst thing is that they are high-fibre carbohydrates. The cellulose in the fibre can't be digested (it goes in one end and out the other) and the starches reduce the body's ability to absorb other vital nutrients such as calcium, magnesium, zinc and iron. A growing number of vets believe that it is the high levels of carbohydrates in modern dog food that are making so many dogs vulnerable to illness and disease.

## *It isn't just the food*

There is, of course, another reason why dogs are becoming overweight: lack of exercise. Society has, of course, become increasingly pressured and many people find themselves without the necessary time or energy to walk their dogs as much as they would wish. Most breeds need a minimum of an hour a day, but the PFMA says that only about a third of dogs are receiving this level. There is another problem, too. In the old days dogs were allowed to roam relatively freely. Even where this was against the local authority's regulations, a blind eye would be turned to the practice of turning dogs out for part or all of the day. My memory may be faulty, but I had no sense growing up that there were more cases of dogs biting people than there are now. Rather, I remember a society that was much more dog friendly. A society in which dogs frequently exercised themselves. I am not suggesting we turn the clock back, but it is another reason why dogs are more likely to be overweight.

### CHECK FOR UNDERLYING HEALTH ISSUES

**If you feel that your dog's weight issues can't be properly explained by diet or lack of exercise then I would urge you to talk to your vet about whether it could be caused by thyroid issues or some type of hormonal problem.**

# 4.
# THE LUCKY DOG DIET!

THE LUCKY DOG DIET!

## FOUR

In this chapter I explain how the Lucky Dog Diet works and provide all the information you need to transform your dog's weight.

### The benefits of the Lucky Dog Diet

The Lucky Dog Diet is everything you could want from a diet.

*It is easy to prepare*
To prepare the Lucky Dog Diet usually takes two or three minutes, once or twice a day.

*The ingredients are easy to find*
It makes use of readily obtainable ingredients. Everything you need can be found in your local supermarket and/or butcher.

*Your dog will go crazy for it*
Dogs love the taste and texture of the diet. You'll be making someone (with four paws) very happy!

*It is approved by vets*
The Lucky Dog Diet has been checked and approved by a number of vets as being safe and effective. See chapter 14 for details and contact information.

*It is easy to understand*
There's nothing complicated about the Lucky Dog Diet. Even the science is easy to understand.

*You can expect rapid results*
Usually you will see a dramatic difference in just 14 days (this is especially true of dogs coming off kibble). We know it is not as if your dog has to get into special clothes (such as a bikini or a morning suit) by a specific date, but still, it is nice to know that it isn't going to take months and months and months to see the improvement.

*Your dog will lose the right sort of weight*
One of the best things about the Lucky Dog Diet is that it leads to the loss of excess fat and not muscle mass.

*Extra exercise is good but not vital*
Although I strongly recommend extra exercise to speed things up and generally improve your dog's health, it isn't vital to the plan.

*It will really improve your dog's health*
In addition to the health benefits associated with being the correct weight, there are all sorts of other health benefits associated with this diet. Indeed, if you continue the diet after your dog's target weight has been achieved you can expect him or her to live a longer, healthier life.

## Backed by research

The Lucky Dog Diet is simplicity itself: a natural diet that is high in protein, low in carbohydrates and contains the optimum level of 'healthy' fat together with an appropriate exercise regime.

Extensive research has been done into the principles underlying the Lucky Dog Diet. Most notably in 2002, a team of scientists published a paper entitled *Weight Loss in Obese Dogs: Evaluation of a High-Protein, Low-Carbohydrate Diet*. Their findings were conclusive: there just isn't a better way for a dog to lose weight.

THE LUCKY DOG DIET!

# *How much should your dog weigh?*

The first step when introducing the Lucky Dog Diet is to work out your dog's ideal weight. What you should be aiming for is 'lean'. That is to say:

- You should be able to feel your dog's ribs when you touch your fingers gently to the rib cage.
- From the side the belly should be tucked up.
- From above your dog should have a proper waist.

The diagram explains this better than words, of course. You will note that the experts believe dogs should have a body condition score of 4.5 or 5 out of 9.

*Under Ideal*
1. All bony prominences evident; no body fat. Obvious loss of muscle mass.
3. Ribs easily palpated. Pelvic bones becoming prominent. Obvious waist.

*Ideal*
5. Ribs palpable without excess fat covering. Waist observed behind ribs when viewed from above. Abdomen tucked up when viewed from side.

*Over Ideal*
7. Heavy fat cover; noticeable deposits over lumbar area and base of tail.
9. Massive fat deposits on neck and limbs. Waist and abdominal tuck absent.

There's no magic formula for working out how many pounds or kilos your dog should be losing. Although it is easy to weigh your dog yourself there is something to be said for getting your vet to do it for you and asking, at the same time, for a target. Another benefit of involving your vet is to check that there are no underlying health issues.

Incidentally, a study by a major dog food manufacturer has shown that a dog's life expectancy is significantly improved by being the correct weight.

## Timing

The beauty of the Lucky Dog Diet is that it isn't really time critical. That is to say, there is no need for you to set yourself the objective of slimming your dog down by a specific amount within a set period. My own experience is that an overweight dog will reach target weight in two to six weeks, whereas an obese dog may require up to 12 weeks (or more) to get into shape. I'd urge you not to rush it.

## The role of exercise

There is absolutely no doubt that exercise plays a key role in weight loss. It is possible for your dog to reach his or her target weight without increasing the amount of exercise taken, but it will slow the whole process down. Moreover, exercise brings with it huge health benefits.

There is a special section, 'Exercise Made Easy', in the next chapter.

## The diet!

From page one of this book I have stressed repeatedly that the perfect diet for your dog uses raw ingredients and is high in natural protein, low in carbohydrates and contains the optimum level of 'healthy' fat.

What does this mean in practice?

You will be feeding your dog ingredients from four different groups:

Group 1: Raw, lean muscle meat and organs
Group 2: Raw, meaty bones
Group 3: Raw vegetables and fruit
Group 4: 'Boosters' such as eggs, sardines &c.

How much of each? Approximately one-third raw meat, one-third raw bones and one-third raw vegetables and fruit. Approximately? Yes! The percentages don't have to be 100% accurate every day, providing you balance things out over a period of a week or two. In the wild dogs eat what is available and receive the nutrition they need over time. They most definitely don't carry scales and calorie counters around with them.

What about the 'boosters' mentioned above? These are to give your dog extra nutrition and vitamins and you simply add one item every other day.

Let me just spell it out again:

- Your dog's diet will consist almost entirely of raw meat, raw bone and raw vegetables/fruit. This is a dog's biologically appropriate diet (think wolf!) and they thrive on it.
- Every meal should consist of roughly 1/3rd raw meat, 1/3rd raw bone and 1/3rd raw vegetables/fruit.
- The proportions are important but you don't have to be obsessive about it.
- You can pick more than one ingredient from each group each day although it is better not to mix protein sources. In other words, serve chicken meat with chicken bones and beef meat with beef bones. However, a bit of mixing and matching is fine if it is easier.
- You'll also be feeding a 'booster' ingredient every other day.

Lists of ingredients (designed to make it easy for you to shop) and sample menus are to be found below.

> An explanation as to why all the ingredients should be served raw is offered in later chapters. In case you have been worrying let me just say here and now that it is 100% safe.

## Stick to less fatty meats

Although your dog needs a certain level of 'good' fat in his or her diet it is important not to overdo it. For this reason, I strongly advise you to avoid fatty meats (such as lamb) and fatty cuts (such as beef with marbling in it).

## How much to serve

Another wonderful feature of the Lucky Dog Diet is that you don't have to concern yourself with the number of calories in the food you are serving.

Instead you simply have to weigh all the food. Initially, I advise anyone new to the Lucky Dog Diet to start by feeding his or her dog 1.5% of its body weight each day (unless it is a miniature or small dog, in which case see below).

Let me give you an example:

> Rex weighs 30 kg.
> Every day he gets 1.5% of his weight in food.
> 1.5% of 30kg is 450g.
> Every day Rex gets 450g of food.

The 450g of food should, of course, consist (more or less) of 1/3rd, 1/3rd, 1/3rd meat (including offal), bone and vegetable/fruit. So 150g raw meat, 150g raw bone and 150g vegetables/fruit.

You can feed it all in one go but I prefer to feed it in two lots as this means the dog will burn up more calories.

## *Should I stick to 1.5%?*

I suggested you begin by feeding 1.5% of your dog's body weight every day but if, after a week or two, you are seeing no appreciable loss in weight then you may need to drop the amount to 1%.

## *Miniature, toy and small breeds need more food!*

Even when they are on a diet miniature, toy and small breeds usually need more than 1.5% of their bodyweight a day. Below are my recommendations. If, after a week or two, you are seeing no appreciable difference in weight then you may need to drop the amount down gradually until you find a level at which your dog is starting to lose those unwanted pounds.

| | |
|---|---|
| 1–2kg | 7% |
| 3–4kg | 5% |
| 5–8kg | 3% |
| 9–10kg | 2% |

I must stress it is always hard to apply hard and fast rules for the smaller dogs. In reality, breeds such as Shih Tzu, Lhasa Apso, Maltese and Bolognese tend to be much more sedentary, so often don't need anything like as much as the normal percentage, even for maintenance, whereas Chihuahuas, Pomeranians, Papillons and Yorkies tend to be more active and ping around all over the place, so burn off food at a much higher rate.

## *How to weigh your dog (and how often to do it)*

Wriggly things, dogs, and they are not always willing to step neatly onto the scales to be weighed. The solution, if you are having a problem weighing them, is to weigh yourself holding your dog and then again not holding your dog. My arithmetic is useless but even I am pretty certain that the difference will represent the weight of your dog.

| Mrs. Smith holding Twiggy in her arms | 93kg |
| Mrs. Smith all by herself | 60kg |
| Twiggy | 33kg |

Ideally, you should weigh your dog once a week and then adjust the daily portion size accordingly keeping it at a steady 1.5% (or whatever percentage you have decided upon).

## *No special equipment needed*

You won't need any special equipment, just a set of kitchen scales, a blender or food processor, a cutting board and knife and a weighing scale (for humans).

## *Preparing the food*

The Lucky Dog Diet requires almost no preparation. Here are some tips.

- When you are serving meat you may like to mince it (if it isn't minced already) or cut it into cubes.
- Dogs are remarkably clever at dealing with carcasses, chicken wings, meaty bones and so forth… it is the most natural food in the world for them.
- The vegetables and fruit can be put through the food mixer and either juiced or grated.
- When you are serving bones just make sure that they are too large to gulp down in a single bite.

Dogs gulp their food because they can't chew and because there are no digestive enzymes in their saliva. So, you shouldn't worry about this. If you want to know more about canine digestion see chapter seven.

A small number of dogs, maybe about one in a hundred, find the switch to raw food a little confusing and they are not quite sure what to do. Tips on helping with this and on preparing and serving their food are to be found in chapter six.

> **Variety is the spice of life. It is important that your dog receives his or her nutrition from lots of different sources. Use meat from different animals. Use different parts of the animal. Use seasonal vegetables.**

## Group 1: Raw, lean muscle meat and organs

Raw, lean muscle meat and organs should make up 1/3rd of your dog's daily food. You'll notice that marrow bones and knuckle ends are included in this group. Why? Because the marrow in the middle of the bone is brim full of (healthy) but high calorie fats.

*On your shopping list:*

Beef heart (aka Ox)
Ox tongue
Tripe
Lean minced or cubed chicken
Chicken hearts
Turkey heart
Lamb heart
Lean minced or cubed turkey
Lean minced or cubed goose
Lean minced or cubed pork
Venison meat
Venison heart
Lean minced or cubed duck
Pork tongue
Beef marrow bones (the knuckle ends are best)

You'll notice that I have left off two easy to obtain ingredients from this list: lamb mince and beef mince. The trouble with any mince is that it tends to have a high proportion of fat in it and this is especially true of lamb and beef. If, however, you can obtain really, really lean lamb or beef it is fine to use it.

## WHAT ABOUT CARCASSES AND WINGS?

Chicken, duck and turkey carcasses (aka 'backs' as in chicken backs) as well as wings can replace both the meat and bone element of the diet depending on how meaty they are. If you can get carcasses/wings then you could feed them as often as three times a week. Unless your dog loves vegetables then you can just forget about the vegetable element on those days.

*On your shopping list*

Chicken carcasses
Chicken wings (remove the skin)
Turkey carcasses
Turkey wings (remove the skin)
Duck carcasses (remove the skin)
Duck wings (remove the skin)
Whole Rabbits gutted, feet removed, beheaded & skinned
Whole Pheasant and other game
Goose carcasses (remove the skin)

## Group 2: Raw meaty bones

Raw, meaty bones should make up 1/3rd of your dog's daily food. I have devoted a whole chapter of this book to the subject of bones so I won't repeat everything here. The important point is that they must be raw (raw bones are surprisingly soft and dogs have such strong stomach acids they can readily digest them). In the wild up to a third of a dog's nutrition (including calcium, magnesium, complex fats and vitamins) may come from bones. Bones keep their teeth and gums clean (it has been proven that dogs with healthy teeth live longer) and exercise their upper body and jaw. Providing the bones are raw (cooked bones can splinter), they are 100% safe for dogs to eat.

*On your shopping list*

- Pork ribs
- Pork trotters
- Venison ribs
- Venison neck
- Chicken necks
- Turkey necks
- Duck necks
- Lamb ribs
- Lamb neck
- Lamb trachea
- Beef trachea

Please remember to read the chapter on feeding raw bones.

## Group 3: Raw vegetables and fruit

Vegetables and fruit should make up 1/3rd of your dog's daily food. It is vital that the ingredients are fresh. Tired looking vegetables and fruit have lost most of their nutritional value. Whether you include one item from this list every day or several doesn't really matter. Unless your dog loves eating vegetables (some do) my advice is to either blend or juice the ingredients and to then mix it in with the other ingredients. Vegetables and fruit are a dog's best protection against cancer. The fruit element should never be more than a small percentage of the vegetable/fruit you serve – say no more than about 10% to 20%.

*Shopping list*

Broccoli
Celery
Celeriac (go easy as it has a high sugar content)
Chinese cabbage
Courgette
Beetroots (go easy as they have a high sugar content)
Carrots (go easy as they have a high sugar content)
Parsnips
Cauliflower
Spinach
Kale
Green leafy vegetables
Butternut squash
Pumpkin
Peppers (red, yellow and orange but not green)
Mangetout
Blueberries
Blackberries
Raspberries
Strawberries
Red watermelon
Apples (go easy as they have a high sugar content)
Pears (go easy as they have a high sugar content)
Bananas (just a small piece and not too often)
Pineapples (go easy as they have a high sugar content)

*Starchy vegetables to avoid: peas, potatoes, sweet potatoes, onion and leek. Fruit to avoid: grapes, avocado, dried fruit*

# Group 4: 'Boosters' such as eggs, sardines &c.

Choose ONE item from this list and add it every other day. In plain English on a Monday you could add an egg, on Tuesday nothing, on Wednesday a few tinned sardines, on Thursday nothing and on Friday a teaspoon of chia seeds. These 'boosters' are not vital to the diet, but help to ensure that your dog receives a wide range of nutrients.

*Shopping list*

Eggs
One egg for a small or medium sized dog. Two eggs for a very large dog. Eggs are packed full of protein and valuable nutrients, essential fats and vitamins. Include shells.

Sardines in water with no salt added
Add one sardine for a small dog, three for a medium sized dog and a whole tin for a large dog. Sardines are a great source of protein, trace minerals and vitamins.

Hempseed oil
One teaspoon. Contains valuable essential fatty acids/Omegas.

Flaxseed oil
One teaspoon. Contains valuable Omegas.

Chia seeds
One teaspoon. Contains valuable amino acids, fibres and minerals. Good source of Omegas, too.

Live yoghurt
One tablespoon for every 10kg your dog weighs. Good probiotic.

## Sample menus

Just to recap. You are feeding your dog 1.5% of its body weight every day (unless there is a reason to vary this amount). The food you serve will consist of 1/3rd meat, 1/3rd bone and 1/3rd vegetable/fruit taken from each of the groups above.

It is better not to mix sources (i.e. serve chicken with chicken). You are weighing your dog once a week and will adjust the quantities as necessary.

Below is a sample menu for a week. You'll notice that on a couple of days I have suggested skipping either the bone or the vegetables. The beauty of the Lucky Dog Diet is that you don't have to follow the rules religiously. There's a bit of flexibility.

# THE LUCKY DOG DIET!

|  | Group 1: Raw, lean muscle meat and organs | Group 2: Raw meaty bones | Group 3: Raw vegetables and fruit | Group 4: 'Boosters' every other day |
|---|---|---|---|---|
| Sunday | Minced chicken | Chicken carcass with no meat on it | Cabbage, broccoli and apple | Egg |
| Monday | Cubed pork | Pork ribs | Carrot and cauliflower | |
| Tuesday | Minced duck | Duck neck | Spinach, mangetout and banana | Sardine |
| Wednesday | Beef knuckle bone | No need for extra bone | Skip for a day | |
| Thursday | Ox heart | Skip for a day | Pumpkin, celery and blueberries | Hempseed oil |
| Friday | Duck back and wings | No need for extra bone | Kale and red pepper | |
| Saturday | Whole rabbit | No need for extra bone | Skip for a day | Live yoghurt |

## *A few words about treats*

A treat is not food. Its purpose is either to reward a dog or, of course, to spoil them! Dogs love receiving treats and we love dispensing them. Of course, a treat is only a treat if the recipient likes it. There are few dogs, for instance, that consider a spinach leaf to be a treat! On the other hand, dogs (like humans) can be trained to enjoy new tastes and sensations. For example, dogs can be trained to view a piece of cut up apple or carrot as something highly desirable.

Here are a few treat tips:

- Size isn't necessarily important when it comes to treats. A tiny, tiny little piece of something desirable (for instance, a piece of cooked chicken quarter the size of a sugar lump) will be well received.
- Little bits of cut up carrot make an excellent treat. If your dog is dubious try cooking them slightly, rubbing them on some meat or adding a few drops of real gravy to give them extra taste. Remember, carrot has a high sugar content, so go easy in terms of quantity.
- Break larger treats into smaller pieces and use more sparingly.
- Air-dried treats (such as air-dried liver) are high in protein but low in fat.
- Avoid rawhide (high in fat) and jerky type (potentially contaminated) treats.
- Apple makes a great treat. Take the same approach as you would with carrot.
- Blueberries (packed full of valuable antioxidants) are easy to carry around and can also be popular.

## An Oscar for Oscar

Your dog may believe, and may even convince you, that he or she is starving to death from lack of food. Don't be fooled. Dogs are incredibly talented actors. In fact, because the Lucky Dog Diet has high quantities of protein and healthy volumes of 'good' fats your dog shouldn't actually feel hungry. A good option, when a dog is making those food eyes at you, is to distract him or her with a game or a cuddle. If you feel you simply must do something then increase the volume of fibrous vegetables in the food. Only be warned: fibrous vegetables can have two side effects: larger volumes of, ahem, waste matter and a greater tendency to, ahem, wind.

# 5.
# EXTRA TIPS AND ADVICE

# TIPS AND ADVICE

## FIVE

The Lucky Dog Diet is, as you can see, absurdly simple and I am willing to guarantee its success if implemented correctly. Below are some of the little wriggles and short cuts I have discovered since I developed the diet, and some facts and other information you may find interesting.

### *A high moisture diet makes dogs happier*

One of the things you'll notice about the Lucky Dog Diet is that the food you serve will be quite moist. This is much healthier for your dog and will have the added advantage of making him or her feel fuller and less hungry. Why does moist food fill a dog up more? Think of the difference between potato crisps (high density, low moisture) and mashed potato (low density, high moisture). You have to eat a lot of crisps to feel full, but much less mashed potato. This is due to the relative moisture content.

### *Exercise made easy*

There is absolutely no doubt that exercise plays a key role in weight loss. It is possible for your dog to reach his or her target weight without increasing the amount of exercise taken, but it will slow the whole process down. Moreover, exercise brings with it huge health benefits. It will strengthen your dog's cardiovascular system and reduce his or her chances of suffering from a range of diseases. Dogs that exercise regularly are happier, too. Here are a few tips:

- Increase the amount of exercise gradually. Your dog will need to adjust to the change in regime.
- If your dog is obese, take it slowly. You don't want to put extra strain on his or her joints.
- If your dog has a short nose (Pugs, Pekinese &c.) don't allow them to get out of breath as their systems can't handle strenuous exercise.
- Exercise comes in many forms – be creative.
- Generally, for a healthy dog, I would recommend an hour a day of vigorous exercise. It is more beneficial if the dog becomes out of breath, since this means his or her cardiovascular system is being exercised.

There are dozens of different and interesting ways to exercise your dog that will make it more fun for them and you. Here are some different ideas:

- Play fetch! Use a tennis ball, frisbee or other toy.
- Treat yourself to one of those snazzy tennis ball launchers.
- Join a flyball club (not suitable for obese dogs).
- Join an agility club (not suitable for obese dogs).
- Make your dog work for every treat (and be mean with the size of reward you give). For example, make him or her go up and down stairs a few times before handing over the reward.
- Swimming is great exercise. There's the sea, rivers and lakes, of course. But also dedicated hydrotherapy and aquatic centres just for dogs.
- Join any sort of training club. Even basic obedience training will burn up the calories.
- Even getting on and off furniture or in and out of a dog bed uses up calories.

Please note it is not advisable to exercise a dog just before or after a meal.

## 'LOOK AT KONG, THE EIGHTH WONDER OF THE WORLD'

This is one of my favourite lines from the 1933 movie *King Kong*. What does it have to do with your dog's weight loss programme? Put a little of his or her food in a Kong (those rubber toy things with holes in them). It will take him or her hours to get the food out, and in the meantime they have been provided with mental stimulation plus they will have used up some calories in the process.

Working on a Kong is quite tiring for a dog and they are more likely to settle afterwards, rather than hanging around the kitchen in a hopeful manner. Make sure the Kong is an appropriate size for the dog. If you have a dog who is brilliant at getting out the food, make it a bit harder by freezing the Kong after stuffing and giving him or her a Kongsicle! take it out of the freezer 10–15 minutes earlier.)

### *Think big! Make the food up in batches and freeze it*

All the food you will be serving as part of the Lucky Dog Diet can be frozen. So, if you would rather not have to shop for your dog every few days, why not make larger batches of the food up, divide it into appropriately sized portions and freeze it?

When I do this I form the food into patties (a bit like hamburger patties) and use plastic sheets to keep them separate in the freezer. You could equally well portion the food into plastic bags, containers or moulds.

Incidentally, bones can be frozen as well. Also, you should never thaw food in a microwave.

Note: there is no health risk associated with freezing food, thawing or partly thawing it, and then freezing it again. This is because modern domestic freezers are so efficient that they bring the food down to minus 18 degrees, or more – quite cold enough to stop most dangerous bacteria from forming. What does happen is that food repeatedly frozen and thawed becomes increasingly mushy and bloody.

## The Lucky Dog Diet promotes the right sort of weight loss

Some research done by one of the processed food manufacturers proved that a high protein diet resulted in fat weight loss rather than muscle weight loss. If food contained 20% protein then 34% of the weight loss was muscle and 66% fat. But by increasing the protein level to 39% the muscle weight loss dropped to 14% and the fat weight loss increased to 86%.

## Water, water, everywhere…

Tap water can contain trace elements of all sorts of contaminants including chlorine, fluoride, arsenic, toxic pesticide residues, heavy metals and so forth. This is not good for humans and definitely not good for dogs. Filtering the water helps. You could also consider rainwater and/or artesian spring water, which tends to be the cleanest and to contain the best range of valuable trace minerals.

TIPS AND ADVICE

## *Please don't support intensive farming*

For the most part farm animals lead short, painful lives in appalling conditions. They are kept indoors, in tiny cages, mutilated and transported hundreds and even thousands of miles before being killed. Furthermore, the way they are slaughtered is invariably drawn out and cruel.

The photographs and imagery used by farmers, producers, food manufacturers, butchers, marketing boards and supermarkets create, by and large, an entirely false impression. Only a tiny percentage of farm animals lead relatively happy and natural existences.

Unless the meat you buy meets certain criteria, the chances are that it has been intensively reared. To buy it is to support cruelty to animals. Of course, it is cheaper than meat from compassionately farmed animals: having a conscience does cost a little bit extra. But if you love animals, it is money well spent. What's more, intensively reared meat is much more likely to be packed with harmful chemicals since intensively farmed animals are given many more drugs to keep them alive.

To ensure that the meat you are buying has not been intensively reared insist that:

Chicken, pork and turkey are free range.
Rabbit and venison are free range or wild.
Lamb and beef have been grass fed or are free range.

If you are buying organic meat, providing it is properly certified, you can be confident that it has been reared with animal welfare in mind.

It is much better for the environment and less wasteful to buy British. It is insane to buy lamb from, say, New Zealand when we have our own here at home. Also, beware of labelling. Ridiculous EU rules allow businesses to buy chickens in, say, Thailand but by cunning means describe them as being British.

If you would like to learn more about intensive farming, you might like to contact: Compassion in World Farming (www.ciwf.org.uk), which was started by an ordinary British farmer; the World Society for the Protection of Animals (www.wspa.org.uk), a leading pressure group; and/or the Soil Association (www.soilassociation.org), the UK's leading campaigner for higher standards of animal welfare.

## The fishy thing about fish

Some experts suggest you incorporate fish into your dog's diet because, in the wild, wolves are, apparently, always holding their paws out to demonstrate how big their catch was and also telling stories about the one that got away.

However, there are various issues surrounding fish as an ingredient. For starters, as it were, overfishing is a massive issue and very few species are unaffected. Then there is the fact that a high percentage of fish contain heavy metals such as mercury and other poisons. In fact, raw saltwater fish often disagrees with dogs. Finally, fish farming does terrible damage to the environment.

I rarely feed fish to my own dogs and we don't sell any fish through Honey's. If you decide to make fish one of the ingredients you feed your dog I would urge you to make sure it comes from a sustainable supply.

## A word of warning about kibble...

Kibble can cause special health issues. Because it is so dry (5% to 10% moisture compared to 70% moisture in a natural diet) and so concentrated, it fails to stimulate the dog's gastrointestinal system. Because of this, it can be dangerous to feed a dog until it feels full. Instead, one must keep the dog constantly hungry.

## Don't let your dog train you

Instead of giving your dog a food reward when they do something cute or for some other reason, try praise: it's just as effective and contains no calories!

## Keep a food diary

A food diary is really useful because it allows you (and your vet, if necessary) to understand how diet is affecting your dog's weight. All you have to do is write down what you feed your dog every day. You could also include a note about how much exercise he or she gets. Involve everyone in the family. If someone slips the dog something forbidden then please, please remember to record it.

## It is all a matter of scale(s)

Please remember to weigh your dog weekly as your dog's weight determines how much food he or she receives every day.

## The pros and cons of green tripe

If there were only one ingredient you could feed your dog, it would have to be green tripe. Nothing else offers such a variety of digestible proteins and your dog would thrive if fed nothing else (although it would still need raw bones, of course). What is green tripe? The dictionary defines it as: 'the raw, unbleached stomach of cattle or other ruminants, after no other treatment than a simple rinse in cold water'. It has a green, fluorescent shine to it, although in colour it tends to be anything from light brown to black.

From a dog's perspective it is almost a wonder food, but from a human's perspective it has a couple of potential drawbacks.

To begin with, it contains a great deal of bacteria, some of which may be harmful to humans (but not dogs). For this reason, it can't be kept in the same fridge or freezer as food for human consumption. It must be handled and served carefully so that no contamination occurs. If you have any cuts or grazes on your skin you shouldn't touch it as it can lead to infection.

Then there is the smell. This is not only strong but also lingers. It's not a bad smell when you get used to it, but it's a devil to wash off and so it really is best to handle tripe using rubber gloves.

In short, it is a nuisance to deal with but well worth the effort if you can be bothered, especially as it is relatively inexpensive.

One final point, bleached tripe is worse than useless as the bleaching process strips out most of the goodness and leaves a potentially harmful chemical residue. Tripe that has been washed in plain water is not as good as green tripe but a less bothersome alternative and can be handled like other meat.

## Reassurance about parasites

The major dog food manufacturers clearly feel threatened by the natural feeding movement and there is definitely a campaign to discredit raw feeding. As part of this campaign it is sometimes suggested that there are dangerous parasites in raw meat. This is incorrect.

One of the reasons why you don't have to be afraid of 'killer' parasites in a 'prey' animal being transferred to a 'predator' is that if this happened all predators would have become extinct long ago! Wolves simply wouldn't have survived. Also, one has to remember that, in the wild, carnivores frequently target sick and old animals as they are easier to catch and kill.

So, not only is it safe for wolves to eat raw meat, but it is safe for them to eat raw meat from poorly prey.

Another reason not to be concerned is the acidity in a wolf's (or dog's) stomach. This is so strong that few organisms can survive exposure.

The parasites that survive on a herbivore are, by and large, very different from the parasites that attack carnivores. There is one exception to this: tapeworm. These can be caught from fleas found on rabbits; so, if a dog eats a whole rabbit (as opposed to rabbit meat), there is a risk. This won't affect you, though, unless you are giving your dog whole rabbit carcasses.

Incidentally, there is a prejudice against pork, because in the distant past pigs used to carry a parasite called trichinosis. This parasite was eradicated in farmed pork in the UK (and Europe) in the 1960s. If you are still nervous about parasites (which I don't think you need to be) freeze the meat down for an extended period.

## A word about hygiene

Dogs may have stomach acids so strong that they would burn your fingers, but humans don't. Raw food does have bacteria on it that could cause health issues for humans. Keep it separate from the food you are going to eat, thoroughly wash any surface it comes into contact with (including utensils, storage containers and so forth) as well as your hands. Use an anti-bacterial soap or mild disinfectant and/or wear rubber gloves. If you don't want to use harmful chemicals, vinegar is a natural alternative.

## Feeding on the move

The Lucky Dog Diet can pose a bit of a challenge when you are away from home. If you don't have access to a freezer, the best option is to take the food frozen and to keep it as cold as possible. It doesn't actually matter if the meat is a little smelly when served (your dog won't mind!) but after a few days the vegetable element will start to lose its nutritional value. Still, with careful management food should last for up to eight or even nine days in a fridge.

# 6.
# MAKING THE SWITCH TO THE LUCKY DOG DIET

MAKING THE SWITCH

## SIX

'At last! This is the very food I have been longing for. Thank you, thank you.' Most dogs welcome the switch to the Lucky Dog Diet with open paws (and open jaws!) but from time to time (I would guess, maybe, one dog in a hundred) a dog will turn its nose up and generally become sniffy at the change in diet.

Why does this happen? I have found that generally it is the really intelligent dogs from loving homes that are more likely to take a stand-offish attitude to the introduction of the Lucky Dog Diet. My guess is that their hunger for attention is greater than their hunger for food. Being smart, they realise that if they don't eat you'll make a fuss of them and this makes them happy. Sometimes, too, dogs become addicted to the high carbohydrate, high sugar, rancid fat taste of kibble or tinned food (in the same way a child may become addicted to junk food) and they object, on principle, to the move to a healthier option.

Whatever the cause, there is no need to worry, as I explain below.

### *Switching options*

*Be firm*
A dog can go up to a week without food and be none the worse for it. Give your dog a single chance to eat every 24 hours, and if he or she doesn't pounce on it with enthusiasm the moment you put the bowl down, lift it straight back up and wait another day. (Anyway, it is not a good idea to ever leave food down for your dog as snacking puts a strain on their digestive system.) Too soft-hearted for such a firm approach? Keep reading.

## Mixing
Slowly start adding raw food to whatever it is you normally feed, increasing the amount every day until it is 100% raw after one or two weeks. This gives the dog's stomach time to adjust to the change. If the dog is regurgitating the food then, having checked it isn't a medical issue, extend the period over which you make the switch. It doesn't really matter if it takes a month or more.

## Cooking
Take the raw food and cook it in a pan (not a microwave and not the bones). Every day cook it slightly less until it is raw. This gives the dog's stomach time to adjust to the change from sterile, processed food.

## Tripe
Fast for a day and then make the switch immediately, but only feed your dog green tripe to begin with. Dogs find this incredibly easy to digest and it contains all the nutrients they need. (For more information about tripe, see chapter five).

## Dogs and vegetables
Some dogs love vegetables; others don't, and the ones who don't may decline to eat their food for this reason. The solution? Give in to them! Remove vegetable from their diet completely and wait for a week or two before gradually reintroducing it. Another approach is to pour a little real gravy or break an egg over the food before serving it, as this will disguise the taste.

# Other things to watch out for

There are other issues that you should watch out for during the switchover period.

## Itchy 'hot' spots
Itchy hot spots on the dog suggest that the food you are providing is a little too rich in one or more specific proteins.

Vary the protein source (switch to different meats) or increase the fat and/or vegetable content.

*Regurgitation immediately after eating*
Regurgitation immediately after eating is almost always caused by a conditioned reflex. The dog's stomach is expecting the normal food and has prepared the wrong kind of enzymes to digest it. When the new food turns up, the system rejects it. It is quite normal in nature for a dog to eat something, vomit it up and eat it again. It is, of course, up to you whether you allow this. But you shouldn't panic. The solution to this sort of vomiting is, initially, patience and then to use one of the switching options mentioned above.

Incidentally, dogs may also vomit bones because they aren't used to eating them, and some people suspect that dogs vomit a meal that they really enjoyed eating so that they can have the pleasure of eating it again! If you have been feeding the Lucky Dog Diet for a couple of weeks and the dog suddenly vomits, this may be an attempt to rid the body of toxins and is not unusual. Obviously, if your dog is vomiting frequently you should check with your vet that there isn't any serious underlying health problem.

*Soft stools*
You shouldn't panic if your dog's stools are runny. It is probably caused by the change in diet and will pass in a few days. It could also be the result of not enough bone in the diet as it is the bone that tends to make the stools firmer. The solution to runny stools is, initially, patience and then to use one of the switching options mentioned above. You could also increase the bone element of the dog's diet. If your dog seems to have a problem with a particular ingredient try it for two or three days and then drop it and come back to it later.

*A word about canine tummy upsets*
There is a huge difference between soft or runny stools and diarrhoea.

It is normal, when switching diet, for dogs to experience soft or runny stools and it can occur if they aren't eating enough bone. True diarrhoea is virtually liquid – like soup. A reliable remedy (apart from increasing the amount of bone you are feeding) is to give the dog slippery elm. Some people recommend mashed boiled sweet potato (possibly with an egg) to firm up stools. If you are worried, return the dog to the old diet and start again when things have settled down. At what point do you call in a vet? In the case of runny stools don't wait more than a week. In the case of true diarrhoea you probably shouldn't delay more than 24 hours. Incidentally, true diarrhoea is not caused by raw food per se but will almost certainly be the result of either a parasite or gastrointestinal problem. If the latter, all that has happened is that the raw feeding has exposed the underlying problem.

# MAKING THE SWITCH

# 7.
# Why Wolves and Wild Dogs Never Get Fat (Even When There Is Plenty of Food Around)

## A WOLF IN ALL BUT NAME

If you look up dogs in any encyclopaedia you will see that their Latin classification is *Canis lupus familiaris* and that they are a domesticated form of the grey wolf, aka *Canis lupus lupus*.

In other words, they are the same species.

The grey wolf has been in existence for over four million years but domesticated wolves (dogs) have only been around for some 8,000-20,000 years.

Whether humans captured wolves and domesticated them or wolves domesticated themselves is not clear. Possibly a bit of both. What is certain is that from early on we selectively bred dogs with a view to developing certain physical and behavioural traits. Thus, over time, we created hunting dogs, retrieving dogs, guard dogs, companion dogs and so forth.

We may have managed to alter the way dogs look and, to a certain extent, think, but physiologically they haven't changed. There is absolutely no difference (apart from size) between the internal organs and digestive process of a Chihuahua and a grey wolf. This is why they should eat the same diet.

## SEVEN

Why don't wolves and wild dogs ever get fat? In fact, why don't you ever see any fat animals in the wild, even when there is plenty of food around?

There are two reasons.

Firstly, and I know I have already mentioned this a couple of times so a squillion apologies for bringing it up again, every species on earth eats a biologically appropriate diet. This ensures that they receive the energy they need and can achieve optimum health.

Secondly, with the single exception of humans, all species self-regulate the amount of food they eat. This means that they maintain the ideal weight.

When designing the Lucky Dog Diet all I have done is replicate a dog's biologically appropriate diet and worked out how much food they should be eating every day.

To do this, of course, I had to study the canine digestive system. Given that I pretty much slept through biology at school, I was surprised at quite how intriguing canine digestion turned out to be. Indeed, if you love dogs I think you will find what follows fascinating.

## *The secrets of canine digestion revealed*

The bond between humans and dogs is so close that it is easy to forget that, being different species, we have markedly different digestive systems. Dogs actually have the same digestive system as the grey wolf and, therefore, need to eat the same diet. The word 'need' is worth stressing. Every living creature on earth must eat a biologically appropriate diet. Some species have a greater tolerance than others, but no species thrives on an incorrect diet and many become ill and die. It is possible for a species to partially adapt to a new diet. Palaeontologists believe that this change takes at least 100,000 years.

## Meat glorious meat

Dogs are carnivores. True, they can and do eat vegetable matter, but anatomically they are designed to catch, kill and eat prey. As with other predatory mammals, they have powerful muscles relative to their size, fused wrist bones and a cardiovascular system that supports both sprinting and endurance. And a quick look inside their mouth is all it takes to understand why they are really much, much closer to being carnivores than omnivores.

## Your dog's mouth is a bit like a Swiss Army knife

No matter how sweet and innocent a dog may look, the inside of his or her mouth tells a different story. Dogs have four main types of teeth, which are designed to perform different and precise functions: catching and killing prey, tearing off meat, scraping meat off bones, and grabbing, holding and crushing bones. They also work like scissors cutting sinews and muscles. None of these teeth, however, is capable of grinding food. Indeed, if you gently try to move a dog's jaw from side to side (necessary for grinding and chewing) you'll find that it is impossible. A dog's jaw can only move up and down.

## All the action takes place in the stomach

A dog's digestive process starts in its stomach. This differs dramatically from humans. We use our teeth to grind our food and moisten it with saliva containing digestive enzymes so that the digestive process is well in hand by the time we swallow. Dogs, on the other hand, don't have any digestive enzymes in their saliva and even if they did it would be useless because they can't grind their food, owing to having jaws that only open and close. Instead, they gulp their food with a view to getting it to where the action takes place (the stomach) as quickly as possible.

## *What happens when the food arrives?*

The stomach starts to produce digestive enzymes and other chemicals to break it down into small molecules that can be absorbed and used by the body. Some of these enzymes are produced by the pancreas, but many are produced by other small glands in the stomach wall itself. To help the digestive process dogs have extremely strong and corrosive stomach acids. Acidity is measured using something called pH. Neutral is pH 7, but when a dog is digesting food its stomach operates between pH 1 and pH 2. Put in plain English: if you touched the natural acids in a dog's stomach, you would burn your fingers. Another important point in relation to this is that most enzymes are extremely sensitive to pH and won't function in the wrong environment. If a dog eats inappropriate food then its digestive system can't function properly.

## *Dogs have evolved to eat a lot, quite quickly*

Dogs can consume up to 5% of their body weight in an extremely short period. To put this into perspective, it would be like a 10-stone human eating, say, seven pounds of food in a single sitting. The inside of a dog's stomach looks rather like an accordion with lots of folds. It expands when full and its muscles massage the food to ensure that the digestive juices work properly. Once all the digestible pieces of food have been dissolved, the muscles squeeze the now liquid mass into the intestine for the final stage of the process and for the absorption of the nutrients. A dog's stomach is designed to finish digesting one meal before being filled again. This process generally takes longer than for humans, although it very much depends on what the dog has eaten.

## Why dogs should eat a natural diet

Every species should eat what it is biologically designed to eat, in other words what it would eat in the wild or as close to what it would eat as is feasible. Dogs are, essentially, wolves and, as such, are designed to catch, kill and eat prey. They have a markedly different digestive system from humans and shouldn't eat the same diet as us, any more than we should eat the same diet as a cow.

## What dogs eat in the wild

Dogs are carnivores and the primary component of their diet is prey. This could be small animals – mice, voles, rabbits, birds, insects and so forth – or it could be larger prey caught with the help of a pack. Either way, they eat everything – the internal organs, the meat, the bones... the lot. Dogs aren't obligate carnivores like cats. They can and do eat vegetable matter.

Wild dogs will search for rotten fruit and will eat the semi-digested contents of their prey's stomach. Some will dig up vegetables and eat grasses and herbs.

Dogs are also scavengers. They eat the leftovers from every animal that is killed or dies. As Ian Billinghurst, a leading proponent of natural feeding, has pointed out, dogs receive 'valuable nutrients from materials that we humans find totally repugnant. Things like vomit, faeces and decaying flesh.' With regard to the faeces, incidentally, these contain the dead and living bodies of millions upon billions of bacteria. They are an excellent source of protein, essential fatty acids, fat-soluble vitamins, minerals, antioxidants, enzymes and fibre.

Not wanting to dwell on an unpleasant subject, but if you have a dog that is on a processed food diet he or she may be eating

## THE GRAIN PROBLEM

Why shouldn't dogs be fed grain? The answer lies in its effect on the pH balance in their stomachs. Normally (see above) this is quite low (between pH 1 and pH 2) because only with a low pH can dogs digest raw meat and bones. Grain has the effect of elevating the pH level and weakening the stomach acids. Weak stomach acids mean that proper digestion becomes impossible.

This is why dogs fed a lot of grain (and there is a lot of grain in most processed dog food) produce high levels of waste matter. It goes in one end and comes out the other.

If grain is processed in some way (rolled, soaked, heated &c.) dogs can digest a small amount, which is what dog food manufacturers rely upon.

Even so, there is another issue. We humans can eat carbohydrates (such as porridge or pasta), convert them to sugars and store the energy in our bodies to use later on. Dogs have no capacity to do this. Grain (rice, wheat, corn &c.) is much cheaper than meat and easier to process, which is why so much of it is used in manufactured dog food.

faeces in order to try to stay healthy (although if a dog is eating canine or feline faeces it will probably be because they contain the undigested flavourings used to make them palatable).

## *What dogs don't eat in the wild*

Almost as important as what dogs eat in the wild is what they don't eat.

For starters (as it were), they don't necessarily eat every day. Depending on where they live, the season, the size of the pack, the available prey and other factors, they may eat as infrequently as every second or third day or even longer without suffering any ill effect. A healthy dog can go a week without food.

Second, and perhaps more important, they don't eat 'complete' meals. Dogs meet their nutritional requirements over time. They will eat what they need or seek it out if their body is telling them they need it.

This is referred to as the 'balance over time' concept. It is crucial to the way dogs should be fed because there is evidence that dogs fed all the ingredients they need in proportion at every meal suffer increased health problems.

Finally, dogs don't eat grain. They can't digest it properly and, even if they could, they can't convert it into sugar and store it for later use.

## **REDUCE YOUR VET BILLS BY UP TO 85%!**

Mogens Eliasen, in his book *Raw Food for Dogs*, quotes a major Australian study on natural feeding. He points out that 'dogs fed on a natural diet develop a strong immune system that will cause your vet bills to go down, maybe even dramatically'. He goes on to remark that the kennels which switched from feeding kibble to raw food 'experienced a significant reduction in their vet bills' with the average saving being 85%! In other words, where they were spending £100 before, they now only spend £15. As explained elsewhere in this handbook, dogs on a natural diet have also been shown to live on average a third longer.

# 8.
# GIVE A DOG A BONE

GIVE A DOG A BONE

## EIGHT

You can't have failed to notice that an important constituent ingredient in the Lucky Dog Diet is raw bone. Let me explain why.

### *In the wild, dogs eat their prey, bones and all*

In the wild, providing they have a choice, all animals eat what is best for them. For dogs this means small prey or, if hunting in a pack, a share of larger prey. They are thrifty, too. Nothing is wasted and that includes the bones. Initially these are ripped, torn, chewed and sucked to remove all the meat and marrow. Then they are gnawed, crunched and (if small enough) eaten whole.

There has been some fantastically interesting (if gory) research in Australia proving this, in which scientists studied the insides of hundreds of wild dogs (don't even ask). One study was by a chap called S. J. O. Whitehouse (*Australian Wildlife Research* magazine, 1977, 4(2): 145–50); another, by a chap called A. E. Newsome (*Australian Wildlife Research* magazine, 1983, 10(3): 477–86). Hundreds of dogs were examined across a wide geographical area. The results were conclusive not only on the bone issue, by the way, but also on other dietary preferences. No wild dog, for example, ever eats grain.

(Note there is more research available on the same topic, including detailed studies by Neville Buck, who studied a wide range of dogs and wolves at Howletts and Port Lympne Wild Animal Parks in the UK.)

## Bones are packed full of vital nutrients

It is easy to understand why the dog wants the meat and marrow, but what makes the bone itself so desirable? The answer is that bones contain a huge number of nutrients that are vital to your dog's health. These include:

- minerals, including calcium, magnesium and phosphorous
- protein-containing essential amino acids, including lysine
- essential fatty acids
- fat-soluble vitamins (A, D and E)
- blood-forming nutrients (these are in the marrow), including copper and iron.

## Bones keep your dog's teeth and gums healthy

Meaty bones are nature's toothbrushes. They keep your dog's teeth clean and gums healthy. Plaque can't build up and decay is prevented. As a result your dog shouldn't develop any of the nasty oral diseases to which many of those on processed food are prone. It will also mean he or she has sweeter breath.

You may be interested to know that a growing number of vets believe that there is a close connection between oral health and general health. One veterinary dentist who has studied this is Dr Gary Beard, who is based at Auburn University in Alabama. In 1991, he wrote a paper pointing out that heart failure, hepatic compromise, renal failure and other serious diseases in dogs could be a direct result of poor oral hygiene. The same year another US vet, Dr Richard Hamlin, of Ohio State University, proposed that diseases of the heart, liver and lungs could be caused this way.

## *Bones provide great exercise, and help with mental health*

Two further benefits of giving your dog bones should be mentioned:

1. They provide your dog with exercise, strengthening their jaws and upper body.
2. They keep your dog occupied. Dogs that have a bone to chew are happier and calmer.

A word about marrow bones. Dogs love marrow bones – the marrow being the creamy centre in the middle of the bone. The upside of marrow is that it is high in nutritional value; the downside is that it is high in fat. If you are feeding a dog that is trying to lose weight then either scoop the marrow out or choose another type of bone.

## *Some bone feeding tips*

- Dogs love bones from pretty much any animal or bird you care to mention.
- A good bone to start with is a beef marrowbone. Ask the butcher to cut it to the right size for your dog: too large to be swallowed in a single gulp, small enough to handle.
- Carcasses (yes, carcasses!) from chickens, turkeys and ducks are excellent, too.
- Only feed raw bones. When a bone is cooked, it hardens and may splinter.
- Choose bones from young animals. Most bones you obtain from a butcher are bound to be from a younger animal, but it is worth checking. Older animals (and birds) may have harder bones, again more likely to splinter.
- The first time you give your dog a raw bone, stay around to watch. Inexperienced dogs can become overexcited and

there is a slim possibility of choking. For this reason a large, meaty knucklebone is perfect. Lamb bones and especially ribs, although excellent (if fattening), can get caught in the mouth and should only be fed to more experienced dogs. Also, hooves are not a good idea as they can splinter. If your dog always chews all the meat off first then lamb necks need to be treated with caution.

*There are a few instances where bones should be fed with caution or not at all. If a dog has just had stomach or anal gland surgery, you should give bones a miss. Some dogs just can't get on with bones and this needs to be taken into account.*

/ GIVE A DOG A BONE

# 9.
# THE UNPALATABLE TRUTH ABOUT MODERN DOG FOOD

## FROM BAD TO WORSE: SPECIAL DIET FOOD

The same dog manufacturers that are helping to cause weight issues in dogs have the audacity to sell special diet food. The diet food is not, on the whole, so different from the normal food they sell – with one definite exception. It frequently contains a sizable percentage of crude fibre. Crude fibre consists of ingredients that have little or no nutritional value for a dog. It helps to make a dog feel full, albeit temporarily, and has the added advantage (from the manufacturers' perspective) of being extremely inexpensive. Crude fibre goes in one end of a dog and comes out the other!

## NINE

Low in protein, high in carbohydrates and drenched in rancid fat, modern dog food is the primary cause of canine weight gain. True, some dogs don't take enough exercise and others take rather more treats than are perhaps good for them, but the real problem is their diet. In a nutshell (often used as an ingredient, as it happens) modern, processed dog food is having a disastrous effect on our woofers' waistlines.

Of course, if the television commercials, advertisements and labelling are to be believed, modern dog food is the only safe thing to give a dog. It contains nothing but natural goodness, has been scientifically formulated and is endorsed by experts, including vets.

What's more, if your dog is suffering from any particular ailment (including being overweight or obese) there is almost certainly a food designed to put it right. Pet food manufacturers would have it that they are your dog's best friend. Once you learn the truth you may begin to feel otherwise. Indeed, you may conclude that you have been misled and deceived.

### *The law doesn't protect dogs*

There is a considerable volume of British and European legislation controlling the manufacture of dog food but it barely considers the health of the animals eating it. Its real purpose is to protect the human food chain. This quote (the italics are mine), taken from the guidance given to pet food manufacturers, demonstrates how little the government cares:

> For pets, the main part of the risk assessment when setting the maximum permitted levels for *undesirable substances* will generally be the extent to which the animal can tolerate them.

In other words, it is legal to use *undesirable substances* in dog food providing they don't kill the animal immediately.

Another disturbing quote from the same guide refers to ingredients:

> The material of animal origin used by the pet food industry comprises those parts of animals which are either deemed surplus to human consumption or are not normally consumed by people in the UK, and derived from animals inspected and passed as fit for human consumption *prior to slaughter*. Animal material of this nature, which is not intended for human consumption, is classified as *animal by-products* under the EC Regulation.

This innocuous statement allows manufacturers to make their food from so-called *by-products*, that is to say hooves, tails, testicles, ears and other bits of animal. It also authorises them to use ingredients that are not suitable for human consumption. How so? If the *by-products* or meat come from an animal that was fit for human consumption *prior to slaughter*, that's fine. The meat could be a year old and completely rotten for all the legislators care.

The notes about labelling are also revealing:

> The labelling requirements for pet food are less onerous than those for feed for farmed livestock [for humans]. For livestock, the ingredients must be declared individually in descending order by weight, but pet food manufacturers have the option to declare them by category – e.g., 'meat and animal derivatives', 'oils and fats', 'cereals', 'vegetable protein extracts'.

The significance of this is huge, as it allows manufacturers to hide the actual ingredients being used in their dog food.

A good way to understand the dog food industry is to study its history.

Modern dog food was invented by James Spratt, an American living in England, who launched the first complete dog food – a biscuit made of wheat meal, vegetables and blood – in 1860. Almost immediately mill owners saw its potential as a way of selling their by-products (basically floor sweepings) and low-cost meat meal at a much higher price than they would otherwise achieve.

From day one, dog food producers made extravagant claims for their products and paid vets for endorsements. Interestingly, the basic recipe for dried dog food, manufacturers' claims and the marketing methods have barely changed at all in over 150 years.

Ken-L-Ration, the first canned dog food, was launched after the First World War, when oversupply led to horsemeat becoming almost worthless. Demand grew and by the end of the 1960s all but a tiny percentage of dogs living in developed nations came to be fed on manufactured dog food. Perhaps this isn't surprising when one thinks how consumers moved from old-fashioned cooking to modern convenience foods.

## A licence to print money

It isn't just that the legislation doesn't consider canine health; it is entirely skewed in the manufacturers' favour. As you can see from the quotes above, they can put in almost any ingredient they want (providing it doesn't actually poison the dog) and can be misleading in what they tell consumers. How did this happen? Since the industry came into being, manufacturers have managed to persuade both the public and legislators that they are experts and can be trusted. They have used clever marketing techniques and veterinary endorsements to great effect and have been much aided by consumer demand for convenience.

It also helps that for many years the industry has been dominated by five multinational corporations, which between them control around 80% of the worldwide market. They are Nestlé (Purina, Bakers &c.), Del Monte (the Heinz range of pet foods), MasterFoods/Mars (Royal Canin, Pedigree &c.), Procter & Gamble (Iams, Eukanuba &c.) and Colgate-Palmolive (Hill's Science Diet, Nature's Best &c.).

These companies lobby hard to ensure that their business interests aren't disturbed by unhelpful legislation. Their biggest single market is the USA, where pet food accounts for $15 billion a year. But the UK market is still sizeable with over £1 billion a year spent on dog food alone.

It isn't just the overall size of the market that makes it so attractive to manufacturers. Processed dog food is incredibly profitable. As one commentator pointed out:

> What most consumers don't realise is that the pet food industry is an extension of the human food and agriculture industries. Pet food provides a convenient way for slaughterhouse offal, grains considered unfit for human consumption and similar waste products to be turned into profit.

## THE UNPALATABLE TRUTH
# Why modern, processed food is so bad for dogs

*Low-quality ingredients*
Modern, processed dog food is generally made using extremely low-quality ingredients. As explained elsewhere in this chapter, that means animal by-products and derivatives and low-quality grain.

*It has been cooked*
Modern, processed food has been cooked. Cooking alters the food's chemical structure, destroys much of its nutritional value and makes it extremely difficult for a dog to digest. A processed food diet, because it is cooked, forces the pancreas to work harder and to draw other enzymes from the bloodstream. This can leave a dog physically vulnerable because the enzymes in the blood are supposed to be protecting the body, not aiding digestion. A number of medical studies show that the pancreas enlarges on a diet of processed food. An enlarged organ means excessive function. Excessive function can lead to degeneration. It is a similar story when it comes to amino acids. Cooking at high temperatures alters the arrangement of these acids, making half of them unusable by the canine body.

Manufacturers try to persuade consumers that the canine digestive system has altered and can now accommodate cooked and processed food. Palaeontologists estimate that a period of at least 100,000 years is required before evolutionary changes occur within a whole species. The most accepted theories estimate that dogs began their association with humans between 8,000 and 20,000 years ago. They haven't, therefore, had time to adapt to eating cooked food let alone processed food, which has only been around since 1860! In the case of kibble it is also too concentrated and too dry (less than 10% moisture compared to 70% moisture in a natural diet).

*It contains grain*
Grain is used a great deal in modern, processed food as it is inexpensive and gives it bulk. Some food will contain up to 65% grain, although this may not be apparent from the labelling. In the wild less than 1% of a dog's diet will be grain. There is a reason why one rarely sees a dog stalking a wheat or rice field. Complex carbohydrates (grains) that dogs eat just end up in an accumulation of lactic acids. Whereas humans can convert complex carbohydrates into sugars and store them for use later (this is what happens when one eats, say, porridge), dogs can't do either. Most grain in processed dog food ends up going in one end and coming out the other.

*It contains fibre*
Modern, processed food contains a high percentage of fibre, described as 'crude fibre' because it is of such low quality. In most cases the fibre takes the form of peanut hulls, almond shells, empty grain hulls, beet pulp and so forth. None of these things offers any nutritional value to dogs.

*It contains preservatives*
Chemical preservatives are added to keep the food from going off. Where there are no added preservatives, it is either because the food has been heated to such a high temperature that no preservatives are necessary or because the original ingredients already contained sufficient preservatives.

*It contains artificial colouring*
Dried and canned food is usually grey. For this reason food colouring is added to give it a more natural appearance. Many trainers believe that the artificial colouring in dog food is one of the causes of behavioural issues in dogs.

*It contains binders*
In the manufacturing process many of the ingredients in dog food are rendered, that is to say they are heated until they turn into a

liquid. In order to make it look like kibble or 'chunks of meat' chemical binders are added.

*It contains unhealthy fats*
Many commercial dog foods have fat sprayed on them as a way of making them palatable. Fat may also be added to improve nutritional value. The quality of this fat is usually poor. Fat can be recycled from deep fryers in restaurants and tallow that rises from rendering plants. It may be rancid.

## Up to 9 out of 10 canine health issues may be caused by diet

A growing number of vets and nutritionists believe that many if not most of the medical conditions that dogs are being treated for nowadays are a direct result of their diet. Tom Farrington, Honey's Chief Veterinary Surgeon, considers as many as 9 out of 10 canine health issues – everything from relatively minor problems such as bad breath, flatulence, itchiness, allergies and dry skin through to major problems such as cancer, liver disease, heart disease and kidney disease – may be directly related to processed food. As Ian Billinghurst, author of *Give Your Dog a Bone*, says:

> Our dogs' disease problems are increasing on a par with their increasing consumption of processed and cooked foods ... dog food manufacturers take useless waste from the human food industry and sell it as dog food. Why do they bother? Advertising implies that they are there to promote the health of dogs. Their primary concern is in fact profit. The laws which govern dog food production do not require it to promote health, reproduction, growth or longevity.

If one cares about dogs it is very easy to get worked up about the processed dog food industry. It is a scandal waiting to happen. The only difference between this situation and what occurred with tobacco, asbestos, powdered milk formula, fast food and all the other consumer campaigns that have led to major changes is that the victims of the processed dog food industry can't speak for themselves.

## How long will consumers (and their dogs) put up with the lies?

There's an Australian study (quoted by Mogens Eliasen) in which it was demonstrated that a dog's life expectancy increased by 30% when fed a raw, natural diet. Dogs that normally were expected to live until age 12 maintained a healthy life until they were 16 years old. This rather implies that dogs fed a processed food diet are leading shorter lives. Which, in turn, raises the question: how long can manufacturers of harmful processed food get away with their lies?

## What are animal by-products and derivatives?

The term 'animal by-products' refers to heads, hooves, feet, viscera and other animal parts you may prefer not to think about. The term 'animal derivatives' refers to heart, lung, muscle meat, testicles and so forth.

Manufacturers can claim that food is 'organic' and even 'fit for human consumption' but that doesn't mean that the ingredients are of high quality. A lung from an organic cow falls into both these categories but you wouldn't necessarily want to eat it.

## Watch out for 'palatability enhancers'

One leading raw food expert, Mogens Eliasen, warns against another rarely discussed ingredient in processed food, palatability enhancers: "The manufacture of these chemicals is a whole industry on its own, supporting the pet food manufacturers with drugs that both taste good and make the animal addicted to the food, once it gets a taste for it. It is literally no different from giving a teenager cocaine or heroin in order to create a customer for more drugs.

# 10.
# A CHAPTER ABOUT SOMETHING NO ONE LIKES TO MENTION

SOMETHING NO ONE LIKES TO MENTION

## TEN

There's no point in beating about the bush: this chapter is about your dog's poo. Why? Because it is an important indicator of your dog's health.

Before we begin, some good news. Dogs on a raw food diet produce much less excrement, and what little there is of it biodegrades quickly and doesn't smell.

### *Normal? What's normal?*

A normal stool should be soft, yet firm. Its colour will be determined by the dog's diet: anything from a mid-brown to nearly black is usual. The more meat in the diet, the softer and darker it tends to be.

If you want to firm your dog's stools up, the simplest way is to add bone.

It is normal to find a greyish bag of slime around your dog's stool from time to time. This is the old mucous membrane, which the intestine sheds every few months.

It is also normal to see the remains of vegetables in the stool. This is vegetable matter the dog hasn't digested and it helps to stimulate the mechanical function of the intestine.

### *A reason to be firm*

It is important that your dog passes relatively firm (even quite hard) stools on a regular basis. Why? In the area under the tail, dogs have two anal glands. These excrete a particular smell when dogs move their bowels, thus allowing them to mark territory and so identify other dogs.

Dog faeces are normally firm, and the anal glands usually empty when the dog defecates, lubricating the anal opening in the process. When the dog's stools are soft, they may not exert enough pressure on the glands, which then may fail to empty. This may cause discomfort as the full anal gland pushes on the anus. If you see a dog pulling its bottom along the floor it could well be because its anal glands are causing it a problem.

## *Stool guide*

- Very dark or black. This is caused by a high percentage of meat in the diet, especially liver and other offal.
- Greyish. Usually the result of eating grain and/or processed food.
- Light-coloured stool. Especially if greyish, may be caused by a liver or pancreatic problem, so worth consulting your vet.
- Greasy stool. When dogs have a pancreatic problem, they are unable to digest fat efficiently. A greasy, sour-smelling stool may be an indication of an underlying pancreatic issue. Discuss with your vet.
- Foamy stool. Could be an infection in the intestine or colon as a result of undigested fat. Again, you should probably discuss with your vet.
- Very hard stool. If your dog is on a processed food diet then the cause is probably one of the ingredients included to keep the stools firm: it is not unknown for dog food companies to use sawdust for this purpose! If your dog is on a raw food diet, a hard stool is usually the result of a healthy meal of bone.
- Blood in the stool. This may be caused by anything from a parasite (such as a worm) to a stool that is too firm. You should keep a sample (sorry!) to show to your vet. Bear in mind that the blood may not be red. If it is not fresh, it may appear almost black.
- Soft and runny stools. A soft, runny or watery stool is not necessarily anything to worry about unless it lasts for several days

or is combined with other symptoms (such as blood in the stool or vomiting). It is normal for stools to be soft, runny or watery when a dog changes diet or eats something that it doesn't want to digest.

## Why raw food produces so much less waste

Mogens Eliasen, a raw feeding expert, has published information about the volume of stools compared to the volume of food being eaten. Meat, offal and animal fat are almost completely digested. The amount of excrement produced will represent between 2% and 7% of the food being eaten. Fruit and vegetables produce around 30% to 60% waste. Kibble, on the other hand, produces 60% to 80% waste. This is because dogs are able to take a great deal of nutrition from meat, organs and animal fat but not from processed food.

## When to be worried about diarrhoea

If your dog has true diarrhoea for 24 hours or soft stools for more than three days, or if it has diarrhoea one day, normal stools for a few days, and then diarrhoea again until it ends up mostly having diarrhoea, then there may be an underlying health issue and you should consult your vet.

If your dog has diarrhoea together with another symptom, such as blood in the stool, vomiting, fever or a change in behaviour, then you should consult your vet.

## Good news for your garden

Dogs on the Lucky Dog Diet, that is to say naturally fed dogs, produce less excrement and what they produce breaks down quickly. As it has no harmful chemicals in it, it won't damage your lawn. If you feed your dog raw food there will be fewer chemicals in its urine, too. This will mean that the urine is less likely to damage your grass or turn it yellow.

# 11.
# MYTH BUSTER!

# MYTH BUSTER!

## ELEVEN

Because the Lucky Dog Diet involves feeding your dog raw meat and raw bones you may find that some people try to dissuade you from introducing it to your dog.

The arguments you'll hear against raw feeding can be very convincing, especially if supported by vets and other experts.

Below, I look at the most common myths and explain why they don't stack up.

### *Myth one: Dogs aren't wolves*

One of the main reasons why natural feeding makes such sense is that dogs and wolves are the same species, the only difference being that dogs have been domesticated.

It is sometimes suggested that because dogs have been domesticated their physiology and digestive systems have evolved and no longer resemble those of the wolf. Therefore, the argument goes, the idea that they should eat the same diet as wolves (or wild dogs) is wrong.

This line of reasoning falls apart both in the bedroom and on the dissecting table! Wolves and dogs can interbreed. The digestive system of a Chihuahua and the digestive system of a wolf are identical in everything but scale. Yes, dogs may have been eating a certain amount of cooked food for the last 8,000–20,000 years but (a) it has only been a percentage of their diet, (b) it is has only been a percentage of domesticated dogs and (c) it hasn't been long enough for them to change the way their bodies digest and absorb nutrients.

The idea (sometimes suggested) that dogs have adapted to

processed food since it was invented in 1860 is laughable.
It is possible for species to partially adapt to a new diet but
palaeontologists believe that it takes at least 100,000 years and
probably a great deal longer.

## *Myth two: Raw food is home to (dangerous) salmonella*

You can pretty much ignore anything anyone says to you about
the dangers of salmonella poisoning in relation to raw feeding.

Salmonella poses a very, very low risk to humans and an
even lower risk to dogs. It is present in 80% to 85% of all raw
chicken and yet the number of people who actually suffer from
salmonella poisoning is tiny. It is even rarer for a dog to suffer
from it and it is interesting to note that when tests were done
and dogs were fed infected meat only one-third had any evidence
at all of salmonella in their faeces. In other words, the canine
stomach acids (which are strong enough to burn your fingers)
killed the vast majority of it off.

So, what is salmonella? Salmonella is a bacterium that can cause
some unpleasant reactions in our gastrointestinal system, like
vomiting and diarrhoea, and often fever. The attack may last about
a week. There was some interesting research done in the US which
showed that people have a risk of about 0.25% per year of getting
infected with salmonella, and 0.05 ppm (ppm = 'parts per million')
of dying of a salmonella infection. To put this in perspective, this
compares to a yearly risk of 108 ppm for a man (33 ppm for a
woman) getting murdered, about 100 ppm for getting killed in a
car accident and 11 ppm for a person less than 91 years old to die
of influenza or pneumonia.

What chance is there of a human catching it from a dog? Dogs
do not carry salmonella in their saliva or on their skin, not even
after eating 100% salmonella-infected raw food. But, when they
do eat salmonella-infected food, about one-third of them will
show a moderate concentration of salmonella in their faeces – yet

no clinical signs of being sick. The only way a human can catch salmonella from a dog is by, to put it bluntly, eating its you-know-what!

Incidentally, dogs eating a processed food diet are just as likely to have salmonella in their system, as it is easy to pick up in parks and elsewhere.

Human beings have been made paranoid about bacteria. In fact, there are more bacteria on a shopping trolley handle than on a piece of raw chicken.

## Myth three: Raw food contains dangerous parasites

In the wild, dogs will usually go for the easiest prey, often animals that are frail and sick. They also eat meat that is rotten, meat that has been buried for weeks and then dug up and, of course, meat that contains parasites. In all these instances they suffer no, or very few, ill effects.

Nevertheless, it is sometimes argued that raw feeding is dangerous to canine and human health because the meat may contain parasites.

This is incorrect for two reasons. First, the food-borne parasites to which dogs are vulnerable do not pose any risk to humans. Second, a dog's stomach acids are so strong that they destroy almost all known food-borne parasites likely to be of harm to them.

If you are still nervous about parasites (which I don't think you need to be) freeze the meat down for an extended period. This will deal with all but a very few, very rare parasites that are never found in food suitable for human consumption.

## Myth four: Raw fed dogs are at risk from neospora

Neospora is a very interesting issue, especially as it was only discovered relatively recently. There have been lots of studies on its effect in cattle but there is almost no research in relation to dogs. Neospora is a parasite and, so far, it seems to be very prevalent in beef herds: up to 80% of them are infected.

Can it be transmitted from cattle to dogs via meat? If it can, what effect does it have on the dog? Finally, is there any risk to humans? There have been so few cases reported in dogs that there is almost nothing to go on. The dogs that seem most at risk are puppies and dogs with compromised immune systems. It seems to follow the same model as toxoplasmosis and coccidiosis. But there are no properly documented cases of it affecting raw fed dogs. Amongst pro-raw feeding vets, the basic feeling is that if it were a serious risk we would be hearing a lot more about it.

There is no need to worry about this risk, especially as neospora has probably been present in dogs and cattle for hundreds of thousands of years.

## *Myth five: Raw fed dogs are at risk of renal failure*

It has been suggested that feeding a dog bones puts them at risk of renal failure, owing to the high amount of calcium/phosphorous to be found in a natural diet.

Calcium is vital to your dog's health and is the most common mineral in the body. The majority of it (99%) is in the bones, with the rest distributed between other tissues and blood. Calcium has an indispensable role in major bodily functions. It is required for the transmission of nerve impulses. It is required for muscle contraction. It is a vital component in the blood-clotting mechanism. It is the structural component of bones and, hence, is of vital importance in growing animals.

Phosphorous is the other dietary mineral required in a relatively high amount in the diet. About 80% of phosphorus in the body is found in bones and teeth, principally as apatite salts and as calcium phosphate. It is located in every cell of the body. Phosphorus is also intimately involved in the acid base buffer system of blood and other bodily fluids, as a component of cell walls and cell contents as phospholipids, phospho-proteins and nucleic acids.

Chronic signs of deficiency include rickets in young animals and osteomalacia in adults, poor growth and lactation performance, and unsatisfactory fertility. Phosphorous is required at levels slightly less than calcium. Meat or organ meats are relatively high in phosphorous but relatively low in calcium.

It is completely wrong to say that raw feeding, eating bones and meat, causes renal failure! To begin with in a well-balanced raw food diet they will be in the correct proportions. Then there is the fact that raw food has lower levels of phosphorous than most canned or dried food. Plus the idea that a high-protein diet increases the chance of renal failure has been pretty much blown out of the water as rubbish.

## Myth six: Raw fed dogs are at risk of choking on bones

Bones, it is suggested, can cause dogs to choke or may rupture the stomach or intestine. In fact, dogs are more than capable of digesting raw, uncooked bones. This is thanks to their strong stomach acids. They are much more likely to choke on dried, processed food, which usually has a water content of between 5% and 10%, far below the 70% water content of a natural diet.

## Myth seven: Raw food is covered in bacteria

Yes, it is! But dogs are surprisingly well equipped to deal with bacteria. Their saliva contains lysozyme, an enzyme that destroys harmful bacteria. Their short digestive tract is designed to push through food and bacteria quickly without giving bacteria time to colonise. The extremely acidic environment in the gut is also a good bacteria colonisation deterrent.

Incidentally, processed dog food is as much of a risk in terms of bacteria as this quote proves: 'Pet foods, commercial or homemade, provide an ideal environment for bacterial proliferation' (LeJuene, J. T. and D. D. Hancock. 2001. Public health concerns associated with feeding raw meat diets to dogs. *Journal of the American Veterinary Medical Association* 219(9): 1224.). The starches, rancid fats and sugars in kibbled foods provide much better food sources for bacteria than the proteins in raw meat do.

# 12.
# WHAT TO DO ONCE YOUR DOG REACHES HIS OR HER TARGET WEIGHT

## ON REACHING TARGET WEIGHT

## TWELVE

The Lucky Dog Diet is the single most effective way I have found to help overweight and obese dogs lose those unwanted pounds (or, if you have a metric dog on your paws, kilograms).

Once your dog has reached his or her target weight, what should you do?

Obviously, you don't want to return to the food that caused the problem in the first place.

Instead, my strong recommendation is to stick with the Lucky Dog Diet but to make a few small adjustments, as described below.

### *Don't rush it*

My suggestion is that you allow your dog to get a little thinner than you feel he or she should be. Not much, just enough to give you a bit of wriggle room, as it were.

Don't rush to change the choice of ingredients or the volume you serve, either. Rather, you should gradually make the changes I am proposing below.

### *Consider different ingredients*

While you have been turning your dog into a new, thinner, altogether happier hound such delicacies as minced beef, lamb and chicken skin will have been off the menu because they all contain higher levels of fat.

Once your dog has reached his or her target weight you can slowly start to introduce a wider range of ingredients, such as:

Minced beef
Minced lamb
Chicken wings with the skin on
Turkey wings with the skin on

## *Switch to 'maintenance' portions*

You have been giving your dog slightly less food than he or she needs, which is why his or her weight has been dropping.

Now you can start to feed very slightly more.

You'll find, after a while, that you can adjust the portion size entirely by feel and without reference to the bathroom scales. Indeed, lots of successful raw feeders simply watch their dogs carefully and adjust the quantity as they go.

There is no hard-and-fast rule but for a dog over 10kg roughly 2% of their body weight in food (including edible bones) every day should be about right for a maintenance diet. In other words, a 20kg dog should be eating roughly 400g.

If you have a working dog, an underweight dog or a dog that exercises a great deal then up this amount to between 2% and 5% of body weight per day.

If you have an elderly or overweight dog then reduce the amount to between 1% and 2% of bodyweight per day.

You can serve the food in as many meals as you want and at whatever time, but it should never be left down for the dog to eat when he or she feels like it. You might be interested to know that because wolves exercise so much they need about three times as much food as a typical dog.

For dogs under 11kg in weight try:

1–2kg: 10% of bodyweight
3–4kg: 7% of bodyweight
5–8kg: 5% of bodyweight
9–10kg: 3% of bodyweight
11kg+: 2% of bodyweight

## Why fasting is good for your dog's health

From start to finish it can take a dog anything up to 20 hours to digest a full meal, a full meal being the amount it can fit in its stomach at a single sitting. This is a very long time when compared to humans, who eat much smaller meals and digest them much faster. Why is the time it takes a dog to digest important? Because a dog's digestive system needs to rest for periods to operate at optimum efficiency. More than this, if the system doesn't get a chance to rest it can be harmful to the dog's health (it needs the time for its liver to transform fat to glucose). My advice is to feed your dog once a day, never to leave food down for it (eat it or lose it being the rule) and to fast your dog at least once a week.

## Achieving balance

Just to remind you, dogs don't eat completely balanced meals in the wild, but get the nutrition they need over time. You don't, therefore, have to worry too much about balancing each meal you feed. Rather, you should be thinking about the balance over a week or even a month.

## What to say to your butcher

It is definitely worth finding a good butcher as it will save you a great deal of time and money. Also, if you live anywhere near a slaughterhouse then see if they can supply you. Either way, it is much, much easier if you have plenty of freezer space.

When searching for a butcher, explain what you are doing and ask for:

scraps
mince (this should be 'visually lean')

inexpensive cuts
offal (heart, kidneys and liver)
raw, meaty bones
chicken, turkey, duck, pheasant and other carcasses.

With regard to the scraps and the mince, it is fine for it to have some fat in it, but it shouldn't be too fatty (more than 15% fat would be a problem). So far as inexpensive cuts are concerned, every butcher has his own ideas what these might be. Take 'skirt', which is the diaphragm under the ribs. Some butchers sell this for next to nothing; others know that there is good, lean meat to be had there and charge quite a bit for it. An efficient butcher will find you inexpensive ways to feed your dog.

Some people feel it is important that the meat they buy for their dogs is suitable for human consumption. Others don't. The truth is that the dogs are unlikely to mind if it is a bit smelly and you shouldn't be too obsessed with the 'best before' date.

> **If you are looking for a convenient supply of ethically sourced meat and bones try Honey's Real Dog Food.**

## ON REACHING TARGET WEIGHT

# 13.
# SAFE WEIGHT LOSS FOR SICK AND POORLY DOGS

# WHAT YOU'LL FIND IN THIS CHAPTER

## Conditions relating to the digestive system

- Bloat or gastric torsion
- Colitis
- Coprophagia (eating faeces)
- Constipation
- Diarrhoea
- Flatulence
- Inflammatory bowel disease
- Irritable bowel syndrome
- Vomiting
- Prebiotics and probiotics

## The thyroid gland made easy

## Internal conditions

- Addison's disease
- Cushing's syndrome
- Diabetes mellitus
- Exocrine pancreatic insufficiency
- Hepatitis (liver disease)
- Impacted anal glands
- Kidney disease (renal failure)
- Liver shunt
- Pancreatitis
- Kidney stones and other purine problems

## Oral conditions

- Gingivitis
- Halitosis (bad breath)

## Skin conditions

- Alopecia (fur loss)
- Itchy skin
- Paw chewing
- Itchy ears and skin problems caused by allergies

## Other conditions

- Arthritis
- Cancers and tumours
- Discospondylitis
- Elbow dysplasia
- Epilepsy
- Hip dysplasia
- Lafora disease
- Luxating patella
- Osteochondritis dissecans
- Spondylosis
- Von Willebrand disease
- A word about steroids

## THIRTEEN

Only too frequently overweight and obese dogs suffer from health issues. These health issues are often caused by either weight issues or diet. Either way, the Lucky Dog Diet is a safe, effective way not only to return your dog to his or her ideal weight, but also to improve his or her health.

In this chapter you will find a short description of some of the most frequently found canine medical conditions, together with advice on what food, herbs and supplements to give to sufferers.

If the Lucky Dog Diet needs to be adjusted I explain why and how to do it.

There is an extremely close connection between diet and health. Eating the wrong foods can cause all sorts of medical issues, whereas eating the right foods can do much to alleviate (and even cure) a wide range of conditions.

As Hippocrates said: 'Let food be your medicine.'

### *Mostly raw*

With one or two exceptions (primarily where the dog's immune system has been compromised), you will see that a raw food diet is always recommended. This is because raw food is the easiest thing for your dog to digest and supports his or her immune system. Where raw feeding isn't recommended, you should not revert to processed food but simply cook the ingredients in the way prescribed. Processed food is an underlying cause for as many as 9 out of 10 visits to the vet, and this includes expensive, so-called scientifically developed, brands.

## A reminder about water

As mentioned in an earlier chapter, water is treated with a great number of chemicals. Ill dogs are less tolerant of these chemicals, and so it is advisable to find a source of pure, clean water. This could be a mineral water (better from a glass bottle than plastic as plastic bottles left in the sun alter the chemical composition of their contents), rainwater or filtered water.

## Why ill dogs do better on organic food

Intensively reared meat and intensively farmed vegetables, especially those imported from outside Europe, are often grown without the regulatory framework we are used to, and may contain a surprisingly high percentage of unnatural chemicals (everything from growth hormones to nitrates and from steroids to pesticides). Furthermore, meat will include the residue of whatever the animal has been fed. This is particularly relevant in the case of grain-fed livestock and poultry, and grain is especially harmful to dogs. It is better, therefore, to feed organic food to ill dogs.

## Free dietary advice

If you need dietary advice, don't forget it is available, free of charge and without obligation, from Honey's Real Dog Food.

## Conditions relating to the digestive system

*Bloat or gastric torsion*
Since the 1980s, the incidence of bloat (also known as gastric torsion, gastric dilatation-volvulus, or GDV) has increased dramatically. In this condition the stomach twists or flips over on itself and air is trapped. Then any food in the stomach begins to ferment, creating further gases. Later on, circulation to the stomach and spleen are cut off to

the point where the dog may go into shock and die. It seems to affect mature, deep-chested dogs the most, especially larger breeds. The condition is extremely serious and potentially fatal. If you suspect bloat, contact your vet immediately.

For a dog that has suffered and survived bloat, a dry food or kibble diet is definitely not to be recommended. Instead, switch the dog to a raw food diet, which has been shown to improve the chances of preventing a recurrence. After bloat, many dogs lose weight and it is important to get this back on as soon as possible, since a healthy weight is one of the factors that reduce risk. Having said this, too much fat in the diet can be harmful. Instead, use lean meat and increase the frequency of meals and total volume of food served.

One of the best things to give dogs that have suffered bloat is green tripe. Avoid vegetables as the fermentation process can produce gas.

It is still not entirely clear why so many dogs appear to be getting bloat. One theory is that dry food is the cause. Most cases seem to occur quite late at night (between 9 p.m. and 2 a.m.) and should always be treated as an emergency. Bloat may be related to stress of some type. Interestingly, dogs that appear to be happy are much less prone to this condition.

*Colitis*
Colitis is either acute or chronic inflammation of the colon and the symptoms aren't terribly pleasant. In acute cases expect vomiting, with diarrhoea containing mucous and blood. In chronic cases the dog will frequently try to pass watery, blood-streaked, mucous and putrid stools. The dog may suffer from flatulence and vomiting. There may be weight loss over time. Do not, however, panic when your vet diagnoses colitis, as it is the cause of around half the cases of diarrhoea in dogs and is relatively common and very treatable.

What causes it? Generally speaking, it is the result of eating something unsuitable (perhaps picked up while on a walk), food intolerances or allergies. Other causes can include infection or parasites. Some cases may be stress-related, and there is a possibility of an autoimmune cause.

In terms of treatment there is every reason to continue raw feeding since this is the easiest food for your dog to digest. If there is the possibility of a compromised immune system, lightly cook the meat before serving. Avoid gluten (grains) and dairy products. Use both a prebiotic and a probiotic. A period of fasting may be appropriate.

*Constipation*
Constipation can occur if a dog becomes dehydrated or has too much bone in his or her diet without sufficient fibre. Other rare causes can be too little magnesium and/or too much aluminium in the dog's diet and also nerve degeneration. One of the benefits of a natural diet is that your dog is less likely to become constipated, but if it does become a problem then add more soluble fibre (ripe apple, pears or tinned sardines or pilchards), while cutting back on the bone element. Reduce the number of chicken wings given, if relevant. Incorporating liver or offal into the diet once or twice a week can help.

*Coprophagia (eating faeces)*
Human beings may find coprophagia (the medical term for eating excrement) disgusting, but to a dog it is a perfectly normal part of their diet. It is believed to have various causes:

- The artificial flavouring and appetite stimulants in processed food frequently pass straight through the digestive system without being absorbed into the body. As a result this can give dog (and cat) faeces a very attractive flavour. It is worth noting that dogs fed pineapple sometimes produce less appealing excrement.
- Boredom! This is especially true in the case of younger dogs and those in kennels who may not have enough to occupy them. Regular exercise, companionship and a selection of toys may help.
- A mineral or trace element may be lacking from the diet. Adding offal (liver or kidney) to the dog's diet may provide the missing nutrients. A broad-spectrum supplement for trace minerals such as Dorwest Keeper's Mix may also be of value.
- The intestinal flora may be out of balance, possibly as a result of

a course of antibiotics. This is especially true if dogs are eating bovine and equine faeces (cow and horse poo, in plain English). A course of prebiotics and probiotics is recommended.
- Submissive behaviour within a pack. Less senior members of a pack will eat the Alpha dog's faeces as an ingratiating behaviour. This is a harder problem to solve. A homeopathic remedy may be of great assistance.

Coprophagia can also lead to worms. Worms can also lead to coprophagia. Therefore, treatment against worms is advisable.

*Diarrhoea*
There is a huge difference between soft or runny stools and diarrhoea. There is rarely any need to be concerned about soft or runny stools. Diarrhoea, when switching to a raw diet, is also not uncommon for the first few days. True diarrhoea is virtually liquid (like soup) and movements are frequent. There are lots of different reasons for diarrhoea, including:

- bacterial infection such as salmonella, E. coli, clostridia and campylobacter
- fungal infection
- viral infection such as parvovirus, distemper and coronavirus
- yeast infection such as Candida albicans
- parasites such as worms, coccidia and protozoa
- poison
- tumours
- stress
- malabsorption syndromes.

It is obviously important to establish the cause before treatment can be recommended, and to this end it may be necessary to run blood and/or faeces tests. Depending on the seriousness of the condition, the options are to (a) do nothing, (b) fast the dog for 24 hours and (c) ask your vet for advice. If it continues for more than 24 hours you should consult a vet.

*Tips for dealing with runny stools and diarrhoea:*
1. Feed a natural diet and plenty of pure, clean water.
2. Give some prebiotics (see below) to feed the good bacteria in the stomach.
3. Use a probiotic (but ideally not live yoghurt). See below for details.
4. Try to avoid antibiotics, steroids and anti-inflammatory drugs unless the dog is seriously ill.
5. Try slippery elm or a modest amount of brewer's yeast to aid digestion.
6. Psyllium husk can be added to thicken the stools.
7. Try a remedy such as Ferrum phosphoricum 12× or 6× tissue salt to help slow the diarrhoea and increase absorption.

Please note that gluten, cereals, cereal by-products and modified starch all contribute to canine digestive problems.

*Flatulence*
All dogs, regardless of their diet, are likely to have a certain amount of flatulence. The most frequent cause is the carbohydrates in processed food – easily remedied by a switch to natural feeding. Antibiotics may also be responsible, in which case a course of probiotics will often help. A small percentage of dogs produce wind as a result of eating vegetables, or particular vegetables, and this can be dealt with by reducing the percentage of vegetables being served or excluding them completely. Incorporating more chicken wings in the diet can help, and so can adding a human-grade organic bone meal supplement.

*Inflammatory bowel disease*
Inflammatory bowel disease (IBD) is a relatively new condition in dogs and similar to Crohn's disease in humans. It is a chronic inflammatory intestinal disease that can occur anywhere in the digestive tract, but most commonly involves the small intestine and colon.

What should you watch out for? Recurrent bouts of diarrhoea, that is sometimes watery, explosive, odd-coloured (yellowish), mucous-coated, slimy and often has blood streaks. Vomiting (sometimes blood-tinged) is not unusual and the dog may have abdominal pain with distension to the bowel and abdomen. The stomach may emit gurgling noises. Dogs are often lethargic with weight loss and may have an increase or loss of appetite. As these symptoms are similar to other conditions it can be difficult to make a positive diagnosis.

In terms of treatment there is every reason to continue raw feeding, since this is the easiest food for your dog to digest. However, reduce the fat content, avoid all grains and dairy products and increase the amount of fibre, such as psyllium husk. Slippery elm can help, too. Use both a prebiotic and a probiotic.

*Irritable bowel syndrome*

Irritable bowel syndrome (IBS) is difficult to diagnose because so many of the symptoms, which may be intermittent, are shared with other conditions. You should watch out for intermittent bouts of diarrhoea or soft stools, increased frequency of defecation, small stools, straining to defecate, abdominal distension (bloating), flatulence, weight loss and, sometimes, vomiting. The stomach may emit gurgling noises. It is believed that diet and stress are the main causes, with some drugs aggravating an already sensitive digestive system.

In terms of treatment there is every reason to continue raw feeding since this is the easiest food for your dog to digest. If there is the possibility of a compromised immune system then lightly cook the food before serving. Avoid gluten (grains) and dairy products. Use both a prebiotic and a probiotic. Slippery elm can be a great help.

*Vomiting*

It is important to remember that dogs regularly regurgitate their food, and this process should not be confused with vomiting that is due to a potential or underlying health issue.

If a dog vomits repeatedly and/or seems unwell in other ways then it warrants contacting a vet. However, if the dog isn't vomiting repeatedly and has no other apparent symptoms, you may like to start by fasting him or her for 24 hours, ensuring that there is an ample supply of pure, clean water available throughout. If your dog seems to be over drinking or having trouble keeping water down then give him or her a block of ice, which will thaw slowly ensuring a constant but reduced supply of water.

Assuming the dog has stopped vomiting after 24 hours, offer a small, light meal. This can consist of scrambled egg or cooked chicken with a prebiotic and a probiotic. If vomiting doesn't reoccur then towards the end of the second day serve a smaller-than-usual meal of whatever the dog normally eats. Resume your ordinary schedule of feeding on day three.

Note: If vomiting continues or is constant or if it contains blood or if it is in tandem with diarrhoea, consult your vet immediately.

### Prebiotics and probiotics

Dogs, like human beings, have bacteria living in their gut. The bacteria themselves are made up of 'unfriendly' strains that can make the dog ill and 'friendly' strains that keep it well. Normally, the balance is in favour of the 'friendly' bacteria, but sometimes – such as after a course of antibiotics, during stress or through poor diet – the 'unfriendly' bacteria get the upper hand. This is called intestinal dysbiosis, a bacterial imbalance that results in an overgrowth of bad bacteria and yeast. Dysbiosis has been linked to various disorders, including yeast infections, irritable bowel syndrome and rheumatoid arthritis. It is treated by restoring the balance with prebiotics, probiotics and a healthy (natural) diet.

Probiotics are beneficial bacteria that can be found in various foods. When you eat probiotics, you will add these healthy bacteria to your intestinal tract. Common strains include the Lactobacillus and Bifidobacterium families of bacteria. Prebiotics, on the other hand, are non-digestible foods that make their way through our digestive system and help good bacteria grow and flourish. Prebiotics keep beneficial bacteria healthy. Happily, you don't need to buy special canine prebiotics or probiotics, as those designed for humans work perfectly. If you need a prebiotic, try aloe vera or chicory. If you need a probiotic, try one containing Lactobacillus, Acidophilus and/or Bifidus-type bacteria with FOS (fructooligosaccharides). Use the minimum recommended human dose.

## *The thyroid gland made easy*

Why do vets (and doctors for that matter) go on about the connection between the thyroid gland and weight? The thyroid gland is responsible for something called the 'metabolic rate'. In very, very plain English this is the rate at which your body converts food into energy. It achieves this with the aid of a hormone called, with staggering originality, the thyroid hormone (how do they come up with these names?). It is, in turn, stimulated by a thyroid-stimulating hormone from the pituitary gland and requires trace amounts of iodine.

Enough science. The real point is that poor thyroid function can produce all sorts of symptoms including weight gain, lassitude, depression and other behaviour changes. Other symptoms could include dry skin, hair loss, thickening or discoloration of the skin, bacterial skin infections, chronic infections (including ear infections), neck pain and seizures.

What causes the thyroid to act up? It can be a side effect of medication (especially of steroids), exposure to toxins (including vaccines) and lack of exercise. Most dogs develop hypothyroidism (the medical term for all of this) between the ages of 4 and 10. If your dog develops hypothyroidism it is worth asking your vet to also look for underlying adrenal gland stress.

What else should you know? There are a number of ways to measure the thyroid health of your pup through blood tests with 'T' names like free T3, free T4, T3, T4, AAT3, AAT4 and TSH. Should your dog be diagnosed with autoimmune thyroiditis, which is confirmed by elevated AAT3 and AAT4 levels, your dog will probably need to have medication to replace the thyroid hormone for the rest of their life.

Most vets in the UK only test for T4 and TSH in routine bloods and can therefore miss these cases. For this reason I generally recommend a more in-depth blood test. Someone who knows a great deal about this is Jean Dodds at HemoPet (www.hemopet.org ) and if your own vet has trouble making a clear diagnosis I would consider asking for a referral.

Usually by the time your pet has enough auto-antibodies to be measured on a blood test there has been irreparable thyroid damage and synthetic hormone replacement is almost always inevitable. However, if there's no autoimmune disorder present, it may be possible to stimulate the remaining thyroid tissue to begin working again. If your dog's thyroid glands have taken early retirement, which is confirmed by low thyroid levels on blood work, it may be possible to regenerate the thyroid using a more natural form of thyroid replacement such as adding pork or beef thyroid gland to food.

## *Internal conditions*

### Addison's disease

Addison's disease is the opposite of Cushing's syndrome in as much that the adrenal gland does not produce enough corticosteroid. It can be a side effect of the drugs used to treat Cushing's. It is less common than Cushing's and can lead to other health issues.

The adrenal gland secretes several substances that help regulate normal bodily functions. Some of the most important products are glucocorticoids and mineralocorticoids. Glucocorticoids such as cortisol have an effect on sugar, fat and protein metabolism. Mineralocorticoids such as aldosterone help to regulate blood pressure and allow the kidneys to maintain a proper water–salt balance in the body (by helping the kidneys retain sodium and excrete potassium). If the adrenal glands are not functioning properly, and the production level of aldosterone drops, a drop in blood pressure and severe dehydration can occur. Dysfunctioning adrenal glands are the main cause of Addison's disease.

Symptoms include muscle weakness and general lethargy, diarrhoea and vomiting, hyperpigmentation, joint pain, lack of appetite and muscle shivers and tremors. The usual treatment is hormone replacement with drugs such as fludrocortisone.

Diet should be under veterinary supervision. Changes in the health of the patient may require a change of diet and this will only be known if blood is monitored. Avoid vegetables and other foods high in vitamin A (such as carrots, celery and liver), also foods high in potassium (bananas, most meats but especially pork). Raw chicken or turkey are excellent as they have lower potassium levels. Salt will generally have to be added to the diet, but this will depend on the blood analysis. Fresh adrenal gland in the diet can be beneficial as can dehydrated adrenal gland as a supplement. It is important that the patient is not stressed. Some herbal and homeopathic remedies can help to achieve this. Patients may also benefit from a small amount of quinoa or porridge – as well as chia seeds, cottage cheese, tuna, egg, sunflower or pumpkin seeds, raw walnuts and raw almonds. The most important thing is to stabilise salt levels and maintain sodium levels.

## Cushing's syndrome

Cushing's syndrome is an enlargement of the adrenal glands resulting in increased production of adrenocortical hormones. Symptoms increase thirst, appetite and the need to urinate. With time the dog can develop a potbelly and an intolerance to exercise with some cases showing muscle spasms and difficulty bending their legs. The coat becomes dry, hairs fine and the skin thins. Hair loss around the flanks and abdomen can spread to the legs, back and head. The diet has to be easy on the liver and help the thyroid gland. High-fat diets should be avoided and the best recipes to follow are chicken with some offal, rabbit and chicken mixed together, venison or lean beef. In terms of vegetables carrot is excellent (for the beta carotene) and broccoli, garlic and grapefruit seed extract. The best supplement to help the thyroid is kelp or a similar seaweed. For the liver add milk thistle and for the heart (patients are likely to suffer from raised cholesterol) add hawthorn. The addition of fresh adrenal gland and/or dehydrated gland powder can also help stabilise these cases.

The diet and supplements need to be changed radically should the patient slip from Cushing's to Addison's. Other supplements that will help patients with Cushing's include vitamins A and D (cod liver oil), vitamin B6, folic acid, vitamin C, vitamin K, calcium, magnesium, potassium, selenium, brewer's yeast and zinc. However, you should not add extra supplements to the diet without consulting a vet. Herbal and homeopathic vets have much to offer in the treatment.

*Diabetes mellitus*
Diabetes mellitus occurs when the pancreas doesn't produce enough insulin or because cells do not respond to the insulin that is produced. Insulin is required for the body to efficiently use sugars, fats and proteins. The commonest symptoms are increased thirst and urination. Although dogs with diabetes mellitus usually have a good appetite, there may be weight loss. Confusingly, some dogs become obese. In many cases cataracts (cloudy lenses in the eyes) may be the first sign that there is a problem. This disease may occur in conjunction with Cushing's syndrome, urinary tract infections, hypothyroidism, pancreatitis and cancer. The condition is usually diagnosed from a urine or blood test.

A natural raw food diet is excellent, but if you are changing the diet from a high-carbohydrate commercial diet the switch must be made under veterinary supervision.

Carbohydrates and acidity are the two core issues for diabetics. One of the reasons why commercial foods are not good for sufferers is that they usually contain urinary acidifiers. Urinary acidifiers can have the effect of complicating the acidosis most diabetics are already suffering from, and the carbohydrates in the diet just keep the problems coming.

If antibiotics are used as part of conventional treatment then prebiotics and probiotics are recommended. Other supplements that can help control the symptoms of diabetes mellitus include magnesium, fish oil, brewer's yeast, zinc and copper supplements and barley grass powder.

*Exocrine pancreatic insufficiency*
Exocrine pancreatic insufficiency (EPI) is the inability to properly digest food due to a lack of digestive enzymes made by the

pancreas. It affects German Shepherds more than any other breed (about two-thirds of cases). EPI is caused by a progressive loss of the pancreatic cells that make digestive enzymes. It is often not diagnosed until well advanced. Symptoms include weight loss, poor hair coat, flatulence and a voracious appetite. Sufferers may also pass bulky, fatty stools.

In terms of treatment there is every reason to continue raw feeding since this is the easiest food for your dog to digest. The amount of fat consumed should be kept to a minimum: chicken and lean beef are both good. Avoid any food (including cooked vegetables such as carrots and peas) containing a high proportion of sugar as this forces the pancreas to work harder. Digestive enzymes and Tree Barks powder can help. It is important to make sure your dog has plenty of pure, clean water.

*Liver disease (including Hepatitis)*
The liver has five important functions, affecting circulation, excretion of waste products, metabolism, immunological defence and blood formation. There are two types of liver disease: primary and secondary. Primary is caused by a non- or sub-functioning liver; secondary is caused by some other condition, such as bacteria, viral parasites, poisons, toxins or tumours.

The most common symptoms associated with liver disease include loss of appetite, vomiting, abdominal pain, enlarged liver, jaundice, discoloured urine, oedema (swelling), weight loss, photosensitisation (skin disease related to sunlight), poor blood clotting, anaemia and a change in stools (either diarrhoea or constipation). Once the cause has been treated, diet has an important role to play, especially in relation to the carbohydrate, fat, protein, vitamin and mineral content. Raw feeding is ideal. Avoid all dairy and stick to a low-fat diet. Conventional treatment can lead to a compromised immune system, in which case food should be lightly cooked. If antibiotics have been used as part of the treatment then it is advisable to give your dog prebiotics and probiotics.

## Impacted anal glands

Impacted anal glands are an extremely common problem for dogs. The glands are situated either side of the anus and discharge a foul-smelling liquid, which is used for marking territories. They are usually emptied by the passing of stools, or if the animal becomes frightened. If not emptied frequently they become impacted, which leads to infection and possibly an abscess being formed. Many vets feel that the primary cause of this problem is processed dog food.

If your dog licks under their tail a great deal, especially if it causes eczema, or if they drag their bottom along the ground, this could well be an anal gland problem. (However, the same symptoms could also be caused by worms.)

One of the benefits of a natural diet incorporating bone is that it creates small, firm stools, which empty the anal glands as the dog excretes.

## Kidney disease (renal failure)

Kidney disease (or renal failure) is fairly common in dogs, especially those reaching their senior years. It is one of the few conditions where we do not recommend 100% raw feeding. Instead, you should take the same ingredients and parboil with lots of water and extra vegetables (especially green vegetables). The extra vegetables will reduce the level of animal protein. When cooking the meat, heat it until it changes colour and then leave it to finish cooking using its own heat. A supplement called Udo's Beyond Greens will help throughput and to balance out the urea. Add it once the food has cooled and is ready to serve so as not to destroy the nutrients. Where high blood pressure is an issue, test to see whether the calcium, magnesium, potassium and sodium are all in the middle of the normal range. If below this level, add supplements. Cod liver oil, zinc and magnesium are very important dietary additions for patients with high blood pressure. *Solidago* (also called goldenrods) can also be of assistance. See below for more about kidney stones and purine problems.

## Liver shunt

The medical term for liver shunt is portosystemic shunt (PSS). A 'shunt' is a blood vessel that bypasses the liver rather than passing through it. Dogs can be born with the condition or it may be acquired. Small dogs are affected more than larger dogs. Diet has an important role to play in the treatment of liver shunt. Normally, the liver removes ammonia from the bloodstream so when this isn't happening it is important to stop the body from producing ammonia in the first place. This can partly be achieved by a low-protein diet. Adding drugs like lactulose and ursodiol to the diet helps with this problem. Make sure the dog drinks plenty of water in order to avoid dehydration. A low-fat diet is best.

Homeopathic support for the liver can be very helpful and should be done under veterinary supervision. Low-potency organ support remedies such as chelidonium, *Carduus marianus*, *Taraxacum* and *Berberis* are recommended. In some cases adding carbohydrate to the diet in the form of organic porridge oats soaked overnight in water can assist in reducing the protein percentage in the diet. Other suitable carbohydrate additions are polenta and brown rice.

## Pancreatitis

The pancreas is a V-shaped organ located behind the stomach and the first section of the small intestine, known as the duodenum. It performs two main functions: it aids in the metabolism of sugar in the body through the production of insulin and is necessary for the digestion of food by producing pancreatic enzymes. Inflammation of the pancreas is called pancreatitis. The symptoms of the disease are a painful abdomen, abdominal distension, poor appetite, depression, dehydration, vomiting, diarrhoea and yellow, greasy stools. The dog may also look 'hunched up'.

There are various causes of pancreatitis, including certain medications, infections, metabolic disorders (high amounts of lipid or calcium in the blood), trauma and shock. Middle-aged dogs and dogs with diets high in fat and/or carbohydrates seem to be at most risk. It is thought that dogs who suffer from Cushing's disease (hyperadrenocorticism), hyperthyroidism and diabetes may also be at risk.

In terms of treatment there is every reason to continue raw feeding since this is the easiest food for your dog to digest. The amount of fat consumed should be kept to a minimum: chicken and lean beef are both good. Avoid any food (including vegetables such as cooked parsnips and cooked carrots) containing a high proportion of sugar, as this forces the pancreas to work harder.

If the pancreas is totally non-functional or very sub-functional, medical supplements such as enzyme replacements may be necessary. This can be done with conventional enzyme replacements (such as Tryplase or Creon 2000) or herbal supplements (such as Tree Barks Powder from Dorwest Herbs).

Patients may also need antibiotics or steroids as part of a conventional treatment. One problem with conventional treatment is that patients can become immunocompromised as a result of the steroids, meaning that they will be more susceptible to infection even from the relatively normal bacteria in raw food. In such a case the food should be lightly cooked first.

## Kidney stones and the purine problem

If you have a Dalmatian, Beagle, Bulldog, Basset Hound, Cocker Spaniel, Bichon Frise, Miniature Schnauzer, Lhasa Apso, Miniature Poodle, Yorkshire Terrier, Dachshund, Newfoundland, Irish Terrier, Scottish Terrier or Irish Setter then you are probably only too aware that these breeds can have purine metabolism problems.

*What are purines?*
Purines are natural substances found in plant and animal cells that are vital to the chemical structure of genes. High levels of purine can be found in any food group (i.e. vegetables, fruit, meat and fish). Certain foods, such as kidneys, game, yeast, mackerel, herring, sardines and mussels have particularly high levels of purine. Others, such as chicken, beef, lamb and non-acidic fruit, contain lower levels.

When cells die and get recycled in a dog's body the purines in their genetic material also get broken down. Once completely broken down they turn into uric acid, which is important to good health because it serves as an antioxidant that protects blood vessels.

However, sometimes uric acid levels in the blood and other parts of the body can become too high. This happens, for instance, when the kidney isn't functioning properly (as it is the kidney that helps keep blood levels of uric acid balanced) or where there is an excessive breakdown of cells. Although kidneys regulate the amount of purine (excreting what isn't required), it is worth remembering that the cause of the problem lies in the liver where purine metabolism takes place.

*The purine problems in dogs...*
The breeds already mentioned above metabolise purine in a unique way ending up with excess uric acid. This in turn leads to urate stones. Worse, if treated with allopurinol to block enzyme-producing urates, dogs can end up with xanthine stones instead of urate stones.

Urate stones are radiolucent and thus can easily be missed, especially when in the kidneys as X-rays pass right through them, leaving no shadow, unlike other stones. It takes air contrast X-rays to show them up. But this cannot be done in the kidney and the stone cannot be felt in the kidney, either. Even ultrasound can miss them but CT (computerised tomography) scanning can pick them up.

*If you have a Dalmatian*
Dalmatians are one breed that has been particularly prone to urinary stones and if you have a Dalmatian or are interested in why then this site will be of interest: www.thedca.org/ stonecharts.html.

*How can diet help?*
A raw food diet without organ meat and with none of the high-purine vegetables (such as cauliflower, peas, spinach, mushrooms and legumes) is generally excellent as a diet for all breeds with a purine metabolism problem. Commercial and homemade low-purine diets can make the condition worse rather than better.

In compromised dogs a high-fat diet can add to the problems

by increasing urate formation, especially in the kidneys. So if you have a thin dog with a purine problem, consider increasing the frequency and size of meals rather than the fat level and check for hidden stones. I recommend feeding more easily digestible meat protein (chicken, for instance) and to avoid less digestible meats (beef, for instance).

Bear in mind that plenty of pure water is also important. The word 'pure' must be emphasised as some additions to water for purification and sterilisation purposes can change the urine pH or entire body chemistry, triggering crystal formation.

What else? 'Table foods' are out and so is anything with salt in it. With regard to diet, incidentally, this may require the addition of potassium citrates (for preventing calcium oxalate crystals) and sodium bicarbonate (for preventing cystine crystals). Always ensure that the diet does not have excessive amounts of vitamin C (ascorbic acid) added, as it acidifies urine, decreasing the risk of the most common forms of stones but increasing the risk of urates.

Finally, do remember to arrange regular urine checks to ensure that the pH stays alkaline and for the presence of either urate or xanthine crystals.

## *Oral conditions*

### Gingivitis
Gingivitis is an infection of the gums and is often caused by the build-up of plaque on the teeth. Symptoms include bad breath, a sore mouth and consequent loss of appetite. Prevention is better than cure and chewing regularly on bones is to be recommended. There is a close connection between oral health and general health. There is every reason, therefore, to feed a raw diet.

### Halitosis (bad breath)
The most common cause of bad breath is poor diet or poor oral health. The latter could be caused by bacteria, saliva and food particles forming plaque. A worse problem is periodontal disease,

which can lead to gingivitis. Other possible causes include diabetes, kidney disease, gastrointestinal disease and infections in the area around the mouth. Respiratory diseases (for instance a sinus infection) and other oral diseases may be responsible. Finally, one should not rule out something that the dog is eating, such as household waste (or worse!). Obviously, the treatment will depend on the cause. Good dental hygiene can be achieved by chewing regularly on bones. As with gingivitis, there is a close connection between oral health and general health, and there is every reason, therefore, to feed a raw diet.

## *Skin conditions*

*Alopecia (fur loss)*
There are many reasons why dogs may lose their coats. Some of the more common causes are allergies, bacterial, fungal or viral infections, mites and poor diet. Trauma to the skin from scratching, burns or wounds as well as stress and hormonal changes (as seen in Cushing's syndrome) may also be responsible. Dietary advice will depend on the underlying condition. A raw food diet will help, however, as it will rebalance the hormones and may even act as a natural hormone replacement (raw meat contains traces of hormones that dogs would be used to ingesting).

*Itchy ears and skin problems caused by allergies*
Itchiness, ear infections, fur loss and skin problems may be caused by a variety of issues, the most common of which is an allergy to food, grains, fleas, ticks, household chemicals, pollen or something else.

If the problem is a food allergy it could well be the result of eating grain or grain-fed meat (intensively reared beef and chicken are often responsible). Traditionally, vets have treated ear and skin problems of this type with a course of antibiotics and steroids, desensitising injections and creams such as cyclosporine A.

Before treatment can be started, it is important to identify the cause of the allergy. In the case of any food allergy the switch to a natural diet may solve the problem, especially as it will help to support the immune system. If the patient has taken antibiotics, a course of prebiotics and probiotics is recommended. One of the ways in which the body responds to a skin-related allergy is to release histamine and other chemicals. Omega 3 can, sometimes, reduce the effects of histamine. Note that other fatty acids, such as omega 6, can actually worsen some allergies.

*Itchy skin*
Apart from allergies (see above), there are many different reasons why dogs suffer from itchy skin, including mites, demodex and mange. Until the cause is known, it is difficult to recommend a treatment, but the following tips may help:

- Various oils reduce inflammation, including cod liver oil, evening primrose oil and starflower oil.
- Consider adding vitamin C to the diet. At least 1000mg daily and even more if the dog can absorb it without diarrhoea.
- If you are taking a dog off medication, use a broad-spectrum multivitamin that includes magnesium as this will dampen down the side effects.
- If the dog has been given antibiotics, a course of prebiotics and probiotics is recommended.

Homeopathic remedies can be very helpful alongside conventional medicine in these cases.

*Paw chewing*
If your dog is chewing its paws, the first step is to check that there are no foreign bodies, such as eggshell splinters, thorns or glass, present and that he or she hasn't sustained a cut. If the dog is on processed food, the cause may be dietary since grain can produce this symptom. A raw food diet is to be recommended. If the cause is boredom then

giving the dog a bone may solve the problem. If persistent check the dog's urine for a kidney problem. It may also be worth checking for a thyroid problem. Finally, it may be the result of blocked anal sacks or an allergy either to some ingredient in his or her food or even to an environmental factor such as contact with, say, household cleaners or stinging nettles.

## *Other conditions*

*Arthritis*
Depending upon whom you talk to, the terms 'arthritis', 'osteoarthritis' and 'degenerative joint disease' may or may not be used to describe the same thing. Degenerative joint disease is characterised by the loss of the smooth cartilage that covers and protects the ends of the bones in a movable joint. The cartilage has no nerves so when it touches the cartilage of another bone there is no pain. When the cartilage wears away, the bone is exposed and, since bones do have nerves, pain and inflammation are caused by the two ends in a joint touching each other. This is the sign that arthritis is present and will probably be progressive. In degenerative joint disease, small bony projections known as osteophytes form on the bone that is closest to the joint.

Degenerative joint disease can occur as a result of wear and tear on an otherwise normal joint and occurs as the dog ages. Osteoarthritis may also occur as a result of hip dysplasia or elbow dysplasia.

A raw food diet helps arthritis because it is low in carbohydrates. High-carbohydrate diets create an excessively acid bloodstream, decreasing uric acid solubility, which in turn leads to joint pain. Bones are an important part of the diet and should include joint bones for their cartilage content (high in chondroitin sulphate) and the marrow of bones including chicken (chicken bones have lots of glucosamine). Turkey is also a good source and, importantly, much lower in salt than most commercial supplements. Such a diet often does away with the need for such supplements as glucosamine and chondroitin, or lowers the required dose.

Supplements that help arthritic pets include cod liver, evening primrose and star flower oil, vitamin C, green-lipped mussel, turmeric, ginger and boswellia (between 1/16th and 1/8th of a teaspoon only), black treacle (also known as blackstrap molasses) and the herbs devil's and cat's claw.

*Cancers and tumours*
One of the ways in which many cancers and tumours can be starved is to reduce the carbohydrates in the diet to 20% or under. (Bear in mind that many commercial dog foods may contain 60% or more carbohydrates.) The purity of the food – ideally it should be organic – and the water is crucial. The vegetables should be as fresh as possible as after a few days vegetables start to lose their nutritional value. Of the many different supplements that can help cancer patients, vitamin C is perhaps the most important: 1000mg a day (or more) is recommended. Please contact Honey's Real Dog Food if you would like more specific advice.

*Discospondylitis*
Discospondylitis (diskospondylitis or vertebral osteomyelitis) is a bacterial or fungal infection of the vertebrae and the intervertebral discs. The resulting inflammation and swelling along with the bone deformities put pressure on the spinal cord, which runs through the vertebrae. Feed the dog a natural diet. Supplements to consider include vitamin C and zinc. Give the dog a natural probiotic.

*Elbow dysplasia*
Elbow dysplasia is more common in fast-growing larger-breed dogs while they are still puppies. Dogs with elbow dysplasia usually have a limp and may hold the leg out from the body when walking. Some will avoid putting any weight on the leg at all. As many sufferers mature, the symptoms may become less severe. Medication may be needed to reduce pain. Some dogs may need surgery and others will have an altered elbow joint with arthritis from a young age. Feed a raw food diet with plenty of bone such as chicken wings, chicken thighs,

drumsticks, pork ribs and marrow bones. Supplement with oil (fish, evening primrose or hemp oil) and vitamin C. Do not allow the dog to over-exercise.

*Epilepsy*

Epilepsy is a disorder of recurring seizures. Epileptic fits are the result of a sort of short-circuiting of the nerves in the brain, so that many nerves are stimulated at once. This can result in quite violent body spasms. Not all dogs that have seizures are epileptic; fits can happen for a number of reasons. For example, older dogs may have an underlying heart, kidney or liver condition, or there may be a tumour on the brain. This last possibility is, thankfully, not all that common. Traumatic injuries to the head can lead to fits in any age dog, as can infections, such as viral or bacterial ones. Occasionally, poisons, such as slug pellets (metaldehyde), will cause a dog to fit. In any of the above cases it is important to treat the underlying problem, if possible, and so eliminate or control the fits that way.

Diet has an important role to play in the treatment of epilepsy. Meats low in glutamate, such as lamb, are best. Avoid meat from animals that have been fed a grain diet. Avoid rabbit, turkey and oily fish, as all are high in glutamate. Epilepsy is definitely on the rise and the combination of wheat and soy in pet foods may well be responsible. Eggs (again low in glutamate) are a good source of nutrition. In addition to the above, one should try to ensure the diet is free of chemicals (preservatives, taste enhancers, palatability factors, chemical antioxidants and so forth), making organic ingredients ideal. Processed foods are particularly bad for epileptic dogs as they are high in grain and incorporate rancid fats.

*Hip dysplasia*

Hip dysplasia is associated with abnormal joint structure and a laxity in the muscles, connective tissue and ligaments that normally support the joint. As the laxity develops, the head of the femur and socket joint separate. This is known as subluxation. Most dogs are born with normal hips; however, owing to their genetic makeup and possibly other factors, the soft tissues surrounding the joint develop abnormally, causing subluxation that leads to altered gait and/or lameness. One or both hips may be affected. Feed a raw food diet with plenty of bone such as chicken wings, chicken thighs, drumsticks, pork ribs and marrow bones. Supplement with oil (fish, evening primrose or hemp oil) and vitamin C. Do not allow the dog to over-exercise.

### *Lafora disease*

Lafora disease (sometimes called Lafora progressive myoclonic epilepsy) is an inherited form of epilepsy that can occur spontaneously in any breed of dog, but it particularly affects the Miniature Wirehaired Dachshund, Basset Hound and Beagle. There is a website (www.laforadogs.org) which is asking for testing to be done for the breeds at risk so that dogs who are carriers are no longer used for breeding. The same dietary advice as for epilepsy (see above) is recommended.

### *Luxating patella*

Luxating patella only occurs in certain breeds, particularly small dogs with short legs, and describes a process whereby one leg bone jumps out of its socket. When it occurs, the leg locks up with the foot held off the ground. It cannot return to its normal position until the quadriceps muscle relaxes and increases in length. Typically, a small dog will be running and then in mid-stride yelp, hold up the back leg and then continue as if nothing is wrong. After a time, the leg drops back down and is used normally. The lameness is very intermittent and does not seem to worry the dog. A raw food diet is excellent. Ensure plenty of bone. Keep the dog from becoming overweight as this will worsen the symptoms.

### *Osteochondritis dissecans*

Osteochondritis dissecans, or OCD (not obsessive–compulsive disorder!), is a disease of the cartilage which may affect the shoulder, elbow, knee or hock. Some dogs will barely have a limp, while others may not want to put any weight on the affected leg. Lameness can worsen after exercise and improves after resting.

It is caused by many factors, including genetics, trauma, rapid growth and poor nutrition. The conventional treatment is strict rest, an NSAID (non-steroidal anti-inflammatory drug) such as carprofen or surgery to remove the damaged cartilage.

It is important that the dog does not become overweight. Feed a raw food diet. Ensure plenty of bone. Supplements which may help include oil (fish, evening primrose, starflower and/or hemp) and vitamin C.

*Spondylosis*
Spondylosis is a non-infectious fusion or degeneration of the vertebrae. The dog is stiff after getting up, appears to be limping (especially after exercise) or begins snapping or licking the lower back. Occasionally, a bony spur or fusing of the vertebrae will cause loss of bladder control and the dog will become incontinent. Feed the dog a natural diet. Supplements to consider include turmeric, ginger, boswellic acids, cat's claw, devil's claw, green-lipped mussel, cod liver oil and glucosamine. It is important that the dog isn't allowed to jump up.

*Von Willebrand disease*
Von Willebrand disease is a common inherited (or sometimes acquired) bleeding disorder similar to haemophilia in humans. Because of the risk of bleeding not being stopped, these dogs need to be looked after very carefully. As even a tiny scratch can cause a problem, patients should not be given any bones. To compensate for potential blood loss a diet high in iron (such as liver) is recommended perhaps two or three times a week. To compensate for the lack of bones a human-grade bone meal should be added to the food so that the patient receives around 700mg of calcium every day. Fish oil is an anti-inflammatory and will protect the kidneys, so one or two teaspoons (depending on the size of the dog) every day is recommended. (If you can't obtain fish oil then cod liver oil is an alternative, although not quite as effective.)

Aloe vera with cranberry juice can also help to protect the kidneys; give 20–60ml (depending on size of dog) three times a week.

Some sufferers of von Willebrand disease haemorrhage frequently, especially internally, and can develop uremia. Additionally, if the problem is autoimmune, where the body attacks its own clotting factors, then the kidneys operate even less effectively. Diet has an important role to play here, too. If the dog is in the uremic stage then raw chicken is recommended. The dog should be given plenty of fluids to keep the kidneys flushed through.

## A WORD ABOUT STEROIDS

Steroids can produce unpleasant side effects (including lethargy, excessive hunger and excessive thirst) and may even cause diabetic-type syndrome. Before putting your dog on a course of steroids, consider consulting a holistic vet to see what other options are available.

# SAFE WEIGHT LOSS FOR SICK DOGS

**14.**
**THE LUCKY DOG DIET IS APPROVED AND SUPPORTED BY THESE LEADING VETS**

# VET-APPROVED DIET

## FOURTEEN

After I had finished writing up the Lucky Dog Diet I sent the manuscript to a number of vets whose opinion I especially valued. Their comments (and contact details) are to be found below. You can rest assured that the Lucky Dog Diet is approved and supported by leading members of the veterinary profession. Incidentally, if you are ever looking for a good vet please do contact my office as we keep details of vets with natural feeding experience.

### *What vets say about the Lucky Dog Diet*

"I have been a vet for 27 years and this is one of the most important books about canine health I have ever read. It isn't just about how to get your dog to lose weight, it's about how to make your dog as well as it can be."
*Geoff Johnson*

"A very useful little book. If you have been struggling with getting your dog to lose weight this book will help you see a different path. A path that consistently creates happier, healthy dogs."
*Chris Aukland*

"At last, a well written book, which addresses the growing problem of obesity in dogs. Clearly explaining the underlying causes of canine obesity and offering a simple and practical solution, every owner will gain new insights into the impact of diet on every aspect of their dog's life."
*Janet Nutall*

"It doesn't take long to realise the reason feeding as nature intended works is it's what nature intended in the first place. Vicky's book is a great introduction for the beginner and will help you get started on a path you and your dog will never regret."
*Mark Elliot*

"At last, a common-sense, logical look at the increasing problem of obesity in our dogs. Vicky has written a great guide to natural feeding and weight loss in dogs that is easy to understand and to follow."

"Drawing on her enormous experience in this field she explains this approach to diet with humour but also with hard fact. I have encouraged hundreds of dog owners to change their dog's diet to a more natural one, and watched the astounding results of doing so. Not just weight loss, but also a huge return to health on every level. I shall be encouraging all my clients to read this book."
*Jane Keogh*

"What I love about this book is that it tells it as it is. You find out when, if and how to diet your dog in a natural way. I have dieted many dogs using this method, and they truly do lose weight in a healthy way — but there is also so much more information within this book about how to keep your dog happy and healthy, not just slim and trim. My most impressive case following this diet was a labrador that went from 50kg to 32kg in a comfortable six months, having had limited success on commercial food (including commercial diet food). Well done Vicky for getting this out there to the public."
*Tom Farrington*

"Obesity is the number one health issue affecting dogs in the UK. This superb little book is packed with simple, practical and effective advice to help you get the pounds off your pooches, and ensure they stay off."
*Neil Coode*

"I wholeheartedly endorse the diet element of this book (although I have some issues with recommending homeopathic remedies)."
*Jill Matthews*

## Contact information

**Mr Geoff Johnson**
VetMB MA MRCVS VetMFHom RSHom PCH
Wiveliscombe Homeopathic And Homeopathic Vet Surgery,
12 North Street, Wiveliscombe, Somerset, TA4 2JY
T. 01984 624999
E. somersetvet@yahoo.com
W. www.vethomeopath.co.uk

**Mr Chris Aukland**
BVSc VetMFHom MRCVS
Forest Lodge Veterinary Centre, Station Road,
Forest Row, East Sussex, RH18 5DW
T. 01342 824452
E. chris.aukland@medivet.co.uk
W. www.medivet.co.uk/forestrow

**Mark Elliott**
BVSc VetMFHom MRCVS MLIHM PCH DSH RSHom
Mark Elliott and Associates, Madam Green Business Centre,
High Street, Oving, Chichester, West Sussex, PO20 2DD
T. 01243 779111
E. ovingvets@gmail.com
W. www.markelliott.co.uk

**Jane Keogh**
Southfield Veterinary Centre, 1 South Walks, Dorchester,
Dorset, DT1 1DU
T. 01305 262913
E. info@southfieldvet.co.uk / j.keogh5@btinternet.com

**Janet Nuttal**
BVetMed MRCVS VetMFHom
Heathfield Vets, Chimneys, Hailsham Road, Heathfield, East Sussex, TN21 8AD
T. 01435 864422
E. janet.nuttall@heathfieldvets.co.uk
W. www.heathfieldvets.co.uk

**Tom Farrington**
MVB MRCVS VetMFHom
'Allswell', Barley Hill East,
Rosscarbery, Co. Cork,
Ireland
T. +353 (0)23 8848811
E. farrington.vet@gmail.com

**Neil Coode**
BVSc MRCVS VetMFHom
Brookmead Vet Surgery, Horsham Road, Cranleigh, Surrey, GU6 8DL
T. 01483 274242
E. info@brookmead-vets.co.uk
W. www.brookmead-vets.co.uk

**Jill Matthews**
BVMS MRCVS
Thanet Animal Hospital, College Road, Margate, Kent, CT9 5TP
T. 01843 226678
E. enquiries@thanetvets.com
W. www.thanetanimalhospital.co.uk

# VET-APPROVED DIET

# VET-APPROVED DIET

# 15.
# MORE HELP IF YOU NEED IT

# MORE HELP IF YOU NEED IT

## FIFTEEN

This book is based on my own experience feeding several thousand dogs a month using either the Lucky Dog Diet or a variation of it. When I first discovered all about the benefits of natural feeding (and the appalling damage being done by modern, processed food) I was so keen to spread the word that I couldn't decide whether to start a company or a cult. In the end I opted for a company – Honey's Real Dog Food – but I want to stress that the most important thing to me, and my colleagues, is canine health.

For this reason we are happy to provide unlimited advice and support to anyone who is interested in making the switch to a natural diet, even if they never plan to become a customer. We're especially pleased to help those caring for dogs with health issues or who are overweight.

Anyway, if you have any questions not answered in these pages please contact us.

Meanwhile, this final chapter explains what we do at Honey's.

### The first week of the Lucky Dog Diet is free

Before I say another word, I just want to mention our new customer offer. If you are interested in trying our food out for a month we will give you the first week free of charge. Alternatively, new customers can try a smaller quantity of our food with a Half Price Hamper.

### We make feeding a natural diet incredibly easy

At Honey's we make it incredibly easy to feed your dog a natural diet. Our raw, fresh dog food is produced using lean, minced meat (choose from a variety of seasonal recipes including free-range chicken, pork, beef and lamb as well as wild rabbit and other game) and grated vegetables. What about the all-important bone element – so crucial to your dog's health? We grind the bone (so that it can barely be seen) and mix it in. We also supply individual bones in convenient sizes as well as chicken wings, handmade biscuits and treats. I will come back to the subject in a moment, but I want to stress that we are deeply concerned about animal welfare and the environment. To the best of my knowledge, for instance, we are the only dog food producer in the UK that doesn't use any intensively reared meat. Incidentally, if you want to go the DIY route we can also help. See below.

## A very personal approach

One of the first things you'll notice if you decide to feed your dog Honey's is that we take a very personal approach. It isn't just that we want to know your dog's name; we also want to know his or her vital statistics, medical history, lifestyle, preferences and personality. We like a photograph, too, so that we can see what he or she looks like. Armed with the information you provide (together with your feedback), we can adjust the ingredients and quantities on an ongoing basis so as to best meet your dog's needs.

## The ordering process

You can order online or by telephone. After you supply us with your dog's details and preferences, we make up his or her food in our kitchens and freeze it. The next stage is packing and shipping. The food, bones and treats are placed into separate containers and labelled. This is then packed (together with feeding notes) into insulated, recyclable boxes and dispatched to you using an overnight delivery service. Our packaging keeps food cool for up to 48 hours. When the shipment arrives, we ask you to take it out of the box and put it into your freezer.

We suggest that before going to bed every night you simply remove the following day's food from the freezer so that it has a chance to defrost. We ask you to keep us up to date with any changes in your dog's health or lifestyle so that we can adjust his or her diet if necessary. A week before we are due to make up the next month's supply we contact you to check everything we plan meets with your agreement and then we repeat the whole process.

## *Excellent value for money*

It costs much less than you might expect to feed your dog with Honey's. We keep the cost down by dealing direct with our customers (so no profit to retailers or wholesalers). The price is linked to the exact weight of your dog and will be calculated for you as part of the order process. Our policy is to charge less than you would pay for the identical ingredients if you purchased them from an ethical supplier, such as Waitrose, Riverford or Abel & Cole.

## *Our 100% money-back guarantee*

We are proud to say that almost all our customers come to us by word of mouth. In order to ensure that we maintain our reputation for quality, service and integrity we guarantee that your food will arrive in first class condition on the promised date. If you are dissatisfied with the quality of our food simply follow the instructions in the delivery box and we will refund the cost in full and without argument.

## *Never worry about running out*

Assuming you and your dog are happy with Honey's, we will set up a regular order for you so that you never have to worry about running out.

## Our Chief Veterinary Surgeon designs and approves all our food

When you feed your dog Honey's you can rest assured that his or her diet has been designed and approved by our own Chief Veterinary Surgeon, Tom Farrington MVB MRCVS VetMFHom.

Tom is an honours veterinarian, holds an advanced degree in Veterinary Homeopathy, has over 28 years of experience in practice, lectures regularly and is responsible for creating an innovative range of homeopathic remedies called Homeopet (www.homeopet.com).

Tom has been encouraging owners to switch their dogs (and cats) to a raw food diet for over two decades. Since then he has seen the practical benefits in thousands of cases.

Tom is responsible for devising all our formulas. He stipulates which ingredients should be used and in what proportions as well as providing guidance as to what volume of food to be fed each day. Thanks to him, you can be confident that Honey's Real Dog Food provides the right nutritional balance for your dog.

## Free veterinary consultation, without obligation

If you are worried about your dog's health, a change of diet could really make a huge difference. One of our retained vets, veterinary nurses or nutritionists will be delighted to review your dog's health issues and make dietary recommendations. You will be under no obligation to accept their suggestions and no charge will be made. Where our consultant recommends a raw diet (and this isn't automatic, as they are all completely independent), we will happily quote for preparing it for you.

## We are deeply concerned about animal welfare

All the meat we use is free-range and/or organic or (in the case of the game) wild. We are concerned about the welfare of the animals we use to make our food. We know and trust all the farmers we buy from. Our objective is to keep 'dog food miles' to a minimum. We try to source everything from local, ethical farmers. By 'local', we mean as close to our kitchens in Pewsey as possible. When ingredients are hard to source locally we may have to go further afield (up to Wales, for instance). We never, ever source ingredients that are not from mainland Britain. We won't touch factory-farmed animals.

## *All our dog food is suitable for human consumption*

It isn't just that our ingredients must pass the 'suitable for human consumption' test: they must be of the highest quality we can find. We don't buy anything that we wouldn't be happy to cook for our own families.

## *About the business*

Our kitchens are based in the depths of rural Wiltshire and we source our ingredients from small, local suppliers.

Our kitchens and offices are just up the lane from my home in rural Wiltshire. We are a very family-orientated business, which is why you may sometimes hear dogs and children in the background when you call. We aren't a big venture and this allows us to offer a genuinely personal service. In fact, we must be the only dog food company in the world that knows just about every single one of its canine customers by name.

## *We donate 1% of sales to Compassion in World Farming*

We donate 1% of all our sales to Compassion in World Farming (CIWF). This is because we believe that the low standard of farm animal welfare both in the UK and elsewhere is one of the greatest scandals in modern human history. CIWF was founded in 1967 by a

British farmer who became horrified by the development of modern, intensive factory farming. Today it strives peacefully to end all cruel factory-farming practices. Its campaigning has resulted in the EU recognising animals as sentient beings, capable of feeling pain and suffering. It has also secured landmark agreements to outlaw the barren battery cage for egg-laying hens, narrow veal crates and sow stalls across Europe. We like the fact that CIWF generally works with business, not against it.

## Just looking for ethically sourced ingredients?

If you want to prepare your own raw food then we can supply you with a range of ethically sourced raw ingredients along with full instructions.

The choice changes according to the season but generally includes carcasses (chicken, turkey, duck &c.), raw meaty bones, heart (ox, lamb, beef &c.), liver, tripe (washed in water), chicken wings, necks (chicken, turkey &c.) and even sheep heads.

If you are new to raw feeding, we usually recommend that you begin with our made-up food and then, once you have got the hang of it, start to make the switch to doing it yourself. All our raw ingredients are suitable for human consumption.

## Please, please remember we are happy to offer free advice

Our main objective at Honey's is to encourage people to switch their dogs to a natural diet. We will happily help you with free advice, tips and recipes even if there is never, ever any chance that you will become a customer. Please don't hesitate to contact us if you feel we can help you.

## How to get in touch with Honey's

*By telephone*
01672 620 260

*By email*
info@honeysrealdogfood.com

*By post*
Honey's Real Dog Food
Darling's House
1–3 Salisbury Road,
Pewsey,
Wiltshire SN9 5PZ

*Or visit our website*
www.honeysrealdogfood.com

# FURTHER READING

# FURTHER READING

# FURTHER READING

'Outside of a dog,' advised Groucho Marx, 'a book is man's best friend. Inside of a dog it's too dark to read.' Quite where that leaves books about dogs' insides I am not entirely sure, but here are details of my favourites.

### Dr. Becker's Real Food for Healthy Dogs & Cats
*Beth Taylor and Karen Shaw Becker*
A brilliant explanation as to why dogs should be eating a natural diet and lots of recipes.

### Dogs, Diet and Disease
*Caroline Levin*
This book explains how canine metabolism and endocrine functions work in a normal dog. A relatively plain-English guide to your dog's innards.

### Foods Pets Die For: Shocking Facts about Pet Foods
*Ann N. Martin*
The title says it all. Ann Martin exposes the dog food industry for what it is.

### Give Your Dog a Bone
*Dr Ian Billinghurst*
The first popular book to promote the idea of feeding dogs raw food and meaty bones. Its author is considered one of the world's leading experts in the subject.

## Grow Your Pups with Bones
*Dr Ian Billinghurst*
Aimed at breeders, this book contains lots of useful information on feeding pregnant mums, new mums and puppies.

## Honey's Natural Feeding Handbook for Dogs
*Jonathan Self*
Written by my co-founder at Honey's. I cover much of the same ground in this book but if you want a plain-English guide to the subject there isn't a better one.

## Natural Nutrition for Dogs and Cats
*Kathy Schultze*
A comprehensive raw feeding guide. Schultze takes a strong line on certain ingredients (such as dairy and honey) which I am more relaxed about.

## Pottenger's Cats: A Study in Nutrition
*Dr Frances Pottenger*
Dr Pottenger discovered, quite by accident, that cats' health degenerated unless they were fed raw food. In his 10-year study of 900 cats, he found the optimal diet for his cats was two-thirds raw meat and one-third raw milk, plus a little cod liver oil.

## Raw Food for Dogs: The Ultimate Reference for Dog Owners!
*Mogens Eliasen*
Available online. An easy read and packed with useful information and research.

## Raw Meaty Bones: Promote Health
*Tom Lonsdale*
Tom Lonsdale has been fighting a long and bloody battle with the various veterinary professional bodies over canine and feline diet. First class book.

## Raw & Natural Nutrition for Dogs
*Lew Olson*
A plain-English approach to quite complicated subjects (well, complicated if one only just scraped through biology at school).

## Real Food for Dogs and Cats
*Dr Clare Middle*
This book is short and well written and provides a comprehensive and easy-to-understand guide to raw feeding. Contains details of relevant raw feeding research.

## Ruined by Excess: Perfected by Lack. The Paradox of Pet Nutrition
*Richard Patton*
An expert in canine nutrition, Patton provides plenty of scientific evidence to back up his claims that canine health is being ruined by modern dog food.

## Unlocking the Canine Ancestral Diet
*Steve Brown*
This book contains fascinating original research into what dogs would eat in the wild and how best to replicate it using 'domestic' ingredients.

# NOTES

# NOTES